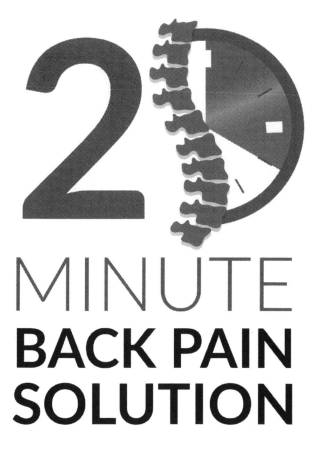

2 MINUTE
BACK PAIN
SOLUTION

Your Guide To Eliminate Back Pain From Your Life!

MICHAEL M. GILBERT, DPT

Dedication

This book is dedicated to all the people who will benefit from reading and applying the instruction within. I have been blessed from my own adversity of back trouble with a seed of equivalent talent to help others overcome their own pain and get back to normal and productive lives. I believe the information within this book will help you. There are many forms of physical treatment out there and I hope this book makes it all easier to understand.

My goal when I became a physical therapist was to help as many people heal naturally from their back pain without the use of drugs, injections, and surgeries. I have been able to do this for the individuals that have come through my clinic. I am excited to be able to help even more people through this book.

I would also like to acknowledge the people in my life who mean the most to me. I am thankful for my wife Adrienne and my children Emily and Alex who have shared in my wins and my losses, pushed me, and encouraged me everyday to become a better man and person in this world. I would also like to thank my parents and family who saw first hand the struggle of my back pain and had to go through that process with me. Without everyone above this book would not have been possible.

To all of my colleagues who have influenced me along the way I say thank you. I have had the pleasure of working with a lot of great people over the years who have molded me into the person I am.

There are too many names to recognize and I wish to recognize broadly so as to not let anyone out. You know who you are, and I say Thank You.

I hope that you enjoy the book!

Table of Contents

Preface

I began my journey to stop back pain 16 years ago. At that time I did not have a Doctorate in Physical Therapy and I was not considered an expert at the treatment of back pain. I had no specific knowledge about the back. I started out as an athletic college bound guy in my freshman year doing everything you would expect a young man to do. I would run, lift weights, play flag football, take classes and do anything else to my body. I was invincible!

Little did I know I had taken my body for granted, and within a few months an onset of pain in my back and down my leg essentially stopped and changed my life. I was a hopeless cause. I was frustrated, tired, and in pain all the time. I had gone from being athletic, active, and on top of my game, to laying around telling friends I could not participate with them and hoping my pain would go away. It took over my life.

I was spending all of my time trying to figure out what to do. I had been to many doctors, took lots of medicines, and got nowhere. It had to stop.

Luckily I was learning about the body through some of my undergraduate courses. I developed a sequence of stretching exercises and decided to start walking daily. I did this every day for the next 3 months. Each day I could see improvement.

Each day I regained flexibility and strength I did not have before. This was not instant. It did not happen overnight. What happened was, I took control of my back pain, and did not allow it to go any further.

The sequence I came up with was not super time intensive, and it was not rocket science. Anyone could have done this. I simply put it together in a logical sequence and made it take a small amount of time I knew I could devote each day. It was the progressive sequence of loosening in the body that I believe helped the most. It was the sequence applied in the same manner, day, after day, after day. When applied with the amount of precision and dedication I had, there was no way I was not going to get better.

I had a tremendous compound effect over time. That journey in life has enabled me to write this book to help YOU. It has been written to be useful at any stage in life. This book is designed as a life long companion in the ever recurring world of back pain. I was relatively young when my back pain occurred. You may be 60 years old and thinking my approach only worked because I was young. I encourage you to read further and allow the next 12 chapters to debunk some of the mental roadblocks that may be preventing you from getting better. Getting past back pain is both mental and physical.

This is not the quick fix...it doesn't exist. Forget about finding the magic bullet and the magic pill. They are not out there. It is about the truth behind the permeant correction of treating the back effectively without drugs and surgery as the main mode of treatment.

The book is empowering. It is about assuming control with a approach proven to work. I am living proof. I have completed this approach, and I continue this approach. I live by this approach. That is how I know it can work for you too.

I have applied these principles with thousands of patients in over ten years of clinical practice. They have been able to witness the changes that can occur in time. I have hundreds of patient success stories on the walls of my physical therapy practice. They are the motivation for this book.

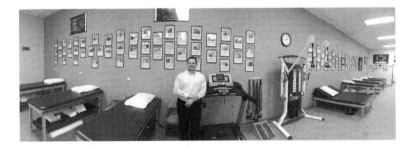

I began my career with the goal in my mind of keeping as many people out of surgery as possible. I feared the prospect of surgery so greatly I wanted to not only stay out of surgery myself, but empower and help others to stay out of surgery as well. This book is the way I can extend my reach beyond the borders of my local practice. If I am truly going to be able to impact as many people as possible I HAD to share my story and let other people know about the methods I used.

The sequence I am sharing with you in this book is also only a small fraction of what physical therapy can do for the back. On a personal level, I am always welcome to treat and help anyone from all over. I can be reached via email for special appointment. If you wish to see me or my team directly, you can email me at **michael.gilbert@gilbertpt.com** and we can set up a time, and arrange details in order to begin treatment.

I consider this book my entry point into your journey through back pain, or maybe your journey through preventing back pain. No matter what, think of me as your guide, as your resource, as your mentor. I am here for you. Refer back to this book often. Refresh your mind when you lose faith, because you will. Refresh your knowledge when you forget the sequence of exercises. Refresh your enthusiasm for sticking with it by reading my story of overcoming back pain. There is hope out there. Reach for it, take it, and succeed you must.

A Challenge was Born:

Throughout this book you will learn about the back, and the way I took control over my back pain and beat it. I am also going to give YOU a challenge. For the next 90 days I challenge you to complete the series of stretching exercises in this book for 20 minutes each day. I am going to offer you the support and information you need. It is contained within the pages of this book. I will even go one step further by having printable stretching guides for use at my website (www.gilbertpt.com).

You can chart your progress, write down notes on your pain to help you understand it better. You can use the Back Pain Elimination daily progress guide to check off your exercises as complete or not. If not, write down what barriers got in your way. Life happens and I know this. You should know that too. Good news is, if we are lucky enough we can to start over again tomorrow and it's a fresh brand new day to make our own. Budget the time in your day just like a financial budget. You make sure your bills get paid right? Make sure your back gets some attention.

If you take the challenge, you are on the path to less back pain. Is there someone else you know who is in pain? Would you like to see them take the challenge as well? Give them a copy of the book and have them complete it with you. Another person going through the journey with you is a sounding board, someone to keep you honest and accountable.

This is a full actionable plan to achieving success. This is not a book that will only give you information. It is both informative as well as a guide. This sequence works. I initially began writing this book without the intention of issuing any challenge at all. The more I thought about it however, I knew I needed to create a need for action. To motivate you to get up and actually take the steps to stop back pain. That was the birth of the challenge. You are 20 minutes a day, for the next 90 days away from less pain in the back. Chapter 10 will be your guide map to success.

I wish you great success and a lot less pain as you take the challenge, so let's get started!!

Chapter One
My Experience with Back Pain

I speak at a great deal of workshops and seminars. At each one I always give the audience a list of my credentials and talk about why I am an expert in the treatment of back pain. This allows everyone to know that I have been trained at one of the best orthopedic Physical Therapy schools in the country and I have completed specialty training in the area of the spine. I have spent countless hours reading the latest research and applying it to the patients I treat in the clinic. All of this information is great and useful, but does it really mean I understand where you are coming from? Can I really FEEL what you are going through sitting in the audience listening to me talk about back pain? Why should you listen to my advice? When you are in pain and you are dealing with it day in and day out you wonder if you are the only one dealing with it. Is there someone out there who understands "My Pain". "I want to see that person!"

This is where my life experience, and physical therapy training come together as one. In addition to being a highly trained expert in the field of treating back pain, I have also been there as a patient.

When I was entering college to begin my journey of learning about the human body I had developed the worst pain I have ever had.

Going into college I was athletic, and had participated in football and track while in high school. The sport of football as everyone knows is quite physical. I played the position of running back. There were many hits to the back and "strange" feelings along the way. I also enjoyed weightlifting and other physical activities. I was what you consider to be an all around active guy.

One day mid-freshman year while in the gym I had been lifting and developed an intense, sharp, stabbing type pain in between the buttock. Every time I bent slightly forward the symptoms would get worse, and it seemed like a great deal of sharp pressure kept increasing. I remember the moment well, I was deadlifting. That was the start. I did not understand what was happening. I had just started school, and we had not even began any coursework that could have helped me understand my symptoms.

So I just kept moving along, it was not THAT bad. A few weeks later the symptoms were still there and the pain moved out into my hip. It still felt like a sharp stabbing pain that was worse with certain movements. I could still get around but it became harder. I popped a few ibuprofen and kept on rolling, after all I was young, athletic, and didn't have time for this pain. As the days and weeks went on the symptoms continued to get worse and I began to stop doing certain activities. I was having trouble sitting in chairs, and starting having a hard time bending forward to put on my socks and shoes. I remember saying "now come on, I'm young, I'm athletic, why can't I shake this." I had no idea what I was dealing with.

After a few months in pain I had finished up my semester and began working my summer job with my Dad doing construction work. This did not go well. Try carrying sheets of drywall with pain in your back and leg. It doesn't work. I had to change jobs and began filing papers at my old high school district office. It was all I could do.

At this point I could not bend down to put my own socks and shoes on, and thankfully it was summer and I could slide into sandals. I had intense pain running from my right buttock down into my right foot. You could trace the pain down the outside of my leg and it felt like a burning, searing sensation. It hurt with sitting, it hurt with bending, it hurt with almost everything. I was taking Advil all day long and was becoming frustrated with the sudden shut down of activity.

At the recommendation of my father I went to see his Chiropractor. I did not know what else to do so I agreed. As a Physical Therapist today I can not believe I did this, but that was then. So I went, and was evaluated. I remember being treated with some manipulation, some electrodes and ultrasound, and hanging on this apparatus I to this day am not sure what it was, and I treat the back! I would limp out, crawl into my van and try to drive home. It was awful. I went a few times without any relief. I was sent for an MRI. Next time in, I was pulled into the office and sat down. He said to me I hate to tell you, but you have 3 large herniated discs in your back and I don't believe you are ever going to play sports and be as active as you would like to be again. I was devastated. It was like being hit by a ton of bricks. "What do you mean?" I was given the card of a surgeon and told I should be consulting with the surgeon to have my back fixed.

After that moment I sat down with my parents and we went to the surgeon. He was a nice guy, well known and respected in his field. He began his exam. I was uncomfortable sitting, standing, laying, nothing was working.

He tested the strength in my right foot. "Hold against my resistance he said." I tried, nothing.

I could not hold my foot up against the resistance. It was as if I had nothing to give, and believe me I was trying. Then he tested my big toe. Again, nothing. The toe was flopping. I could not believe that I had gone from squatting and deadlifting significant weight in the gym to this.

It was confirmation of a large L4-L5 and L5-S1 disc herniation putting pressure on the nerve coming out of the back. After the exam I sat on the table fearful of the advice I was going to hear. I thought I had only one option, surgery. The first thing out of my mouth was "I do not want surgery and I'll do whatever I have to do in order to avoid it." After listening to my plea, he agreed to a course of more medicine, and a series of injections. So there I left with more pills in hand and a referral to a pain management doctor to get an epidural steroid injection.

If you have ever gone through this type of pain, you know that seeing different doctors and being on their waiting lists to be seen is not the quickest of processes. So it was a few weeks and then on to the next doctor. I was going in for the epidural steroid injection. My parents helped drive since I was not sure what to expect. I went in, and laid on the table face down. Looking to the side I talked to the nursing staff who let me watch the screen to see the needle be X-Ray guided into my back. First was just a pinch to numb the area in the low back. Then came the big needle.

It felt like a great deal of pressure going down into the back. I watched the needle go between my vertebrae. As the medicine went in the doctor said "I'll go slow." As he delivered the medicine through the needle it felt as if my leg was blowing up like a balloon and catching fire. It got worse, to the point where I was sure it was going to explode. In hindsight this was the medicine squeezing down on the nerve. It was incredibly intense. Once it ended I was unsure if I was going to be able to move. My leg was on fire, felt like it was blown up like a balloon, and I was still in pain. I limped out of there and crawled into the back of my parents car. I could do nothing but lay flat in the back seat and off we went.

That day I was advised to not move too much, and it was a good thing, *because I couldn't.*

Over the following day the effects of the shot did subside, but my pain was still in the leg and pretty severe. I could move, but I was just a little disappointed that it did not take away all the pain.

The way that epidurals work however in the dosing is to deliver another shot within the next two weeks. So I went in for the next injection. This one felt much better being delivered. I did not have the same feeling of fire and leg exploding as the first one. I came out of the injection, pain was down, but still there. I was frustrated.

The Decision

At this point I knew something needed to change and I had to stop being afraid of the pain and making things worse. I decided that I was going to start performing a series of stretches, walk everyday and begin some very light leg strengthening like I had done before in sports.

I decided on a certain group of stretches, and did it in a certain sequence everyday. It was a shift mentally from victim, to full on attack mode.

I was determined.

I had lost a great deal of weight most of which was muscle (gained undesirable fat!).

I wanted my body back.

I wanted to get my activities back.

I was tired of not being able to participate in the activities I enjoyed.

I was tired of everyone around me treating me like I was a fragile china doll that would break at any given moment.

Our family had a boat and I used to like to tube and wakeboard. I wanted to do this again. I did not want to have to ride in the boat and be afraid of every bump we hit in the water. I wanted to go to the amusement park and not be afraid to ride the roller coaster.

So while it may seem like I just gave you the entire story of my back, this is really where it began. It was at this point where I made the turn from constant pain to constant progress toward where I am today. This book is about that journey and how you too can get there from wherever you are starting from. You may not have as intense of a back problem as I did, or you may be worse. No matter what, you will be able to take the lessons learned in this book and put them into practice in your everyday life to improve your health and eliminate the pain in your back. Do not focus on how far you are away from where you want to be, focus on the tiny steps you need to make to get there. Thank you for allowing me to be your guide. I know that by following this 20 minute back pain solution you will decrease your pain and improve your life. Before we get into the solution itself, we need to lay the foundation for how it works.

CHAPTER 1 KEY POINTS

🔑 Pain can happen at all ages in life

🔑 There needs to be a determination to get better

🔑 Focus small for big results

🔑 Fear should not be your guide

Chapter Two
Why Does My Back Hurt?

The spine is one of the most complex structures in the human body. If you think about it, the spine is the center of the universe in the body. The head, arms, and legs are all connected to it and can be effected by the function of the spine. The spine is made up of 24 main vertebrae that can move and then 9 fused vertebrae that form the sacrum and the coccyx (better known as the tailbone). The spine is separated into 3 main sections. The Cervical, Thoracic, and Lumbar Spine.

The Cervical Spine

This section of the spine has 7 bones. This is the part of the spine that makes up the neck and connects the head to the body. It allows the head to rotate side to side, bend forward, backward, and tilt side to side. It also serves to protect the spinal cord as it comes down off of the brain. The spinal cord is housed within a boney arch and travels within the vertebrae down the body to the lumbar spine. There are also major arteries that travel through the vertebrae and lead up into the brain. These are called the vertebral arteries. The cervical spine can be prone to injuries of overuse, poor posture, whiplash accidents and more. One of the most common areas of pain is where the neck meets the shoulders. Usually people will say something such as "I carry my stress in my neck and shoulders." In the age of computers and tablets and smartphones, the neck is placed in poor positions for longer periods of time than ever before.

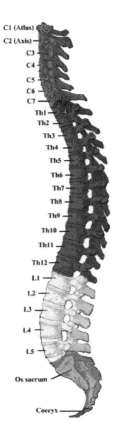

Figure: This is a picture of the cervical spine, the thoracic spine, the lumbar spine and the sacrum/coccyx.

The Thoracic Spine

This section of the spine consists of 12 vertebrae and separates the neck from the lower back. This is the middle section of your body. The thoracic spine also has the ribs which help to protect the vital organs of the body such as the lungs, the heart, the liver, etc. This is an inherently stiff area of the body due to the connection of the ribs to these vertebrae. That is a good thing for we do not want anything to crush our organs.

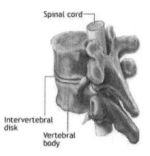

Figure: The above diagram is a picture of a thoracic vertebral segment. It consists of a vertebrae (bone) , then a disc, then another vertebrae (bone) with a corresponding nerve that exits between the two bones.

The thoracic spine can create problems for people in particular who have conditions such as osteoporosis where the structure of the bone can become more brittle and fracture. These are known as compression fractures and they can be quite painful.

Biomechanically we have more and more evidence coming out these days that tie pain that occurs in the neck to the mobility of the thoracic spine. This means that the tighter the thoracic spine, or more rigid it is, the more likely the neck is to become painful and give a person a problem.

The Lumbar Spine

The Lumbar spine is the bottom portion of the back. It is the foundation that effects everything back up the spine. It also effects everything down through the hips and legs. The lumbar spine consists of 5 vertebrae. They are larger vertebrae than in the neck and thoracic spine. The lumbar spine represents 1 in 4 visits to the primary care physician for pain. More than 80% of people are going to experience back pain at some point in there life. It easily represents the single largest condition I treat in my professional practice and I have devoted nearly my entire career to studying the back and treating the pain it produces. To delve deeper into the way the lumbar spine works you need to understand the anatomy.

A lumbar segment represents a few main parts. A vertebrae, a disc, and another vertebrae. There are nerves that exit from the spinal segment through a hole called a foramina. When talking about a disc, they are named for the vertebrae they are between. For example, the disc between the L4 vertebrae and the L5 vertebrae is called L4/5.

There are also two large joints that connect the spine to the pelvic bones called the sacroiliac joints. They can create pain and alter the biomechanics of the entire leg. If the sacroiliac joints are not in the correct position it can influence the back, the hips, the knees and down into the ankles and feet. This can create a snowball effect of injury over time if left untreated and someone who previously did not have a problem at the knee may all of a sudden have a problem. The only reason it started in the first place was because of a pain in the back.

Pain that is present in the lower back can be present at the location of the injury or down the leg. In my field, the biggest component to helping someone effectively treat a back problem is actually determining where it is coming from in the first place. If you can not find an accurate diagnosis, you will not be able to accurately treat the back. Different back problems have different presentations and someone will come in with different complaints. Symptoms may be similar between conditions though. Confused?

Things Happen Over Time

We have just mentioned a little bit of information about the three main areas of the spine. I will go more in depth about conditions of the lumbar spine later in the book (see Chapter 6.). Before that however it is important to understand how problems develop in the spine, and it's really not all that complicated. You have a stack of 24 moving bones sitting on top of 9 fused bones. They are controlled in every way by the muscles that overly them. Muscles connect to the vertebrae at varying points all up and down the spine. Some muscles are large and long and are responsible for big movements of the body. Other muscles are very small and only span a few inches at best. The small muscles are what are called proprioceptors. This means that there main function is to simply help give feedback to the brain about where the body is in space. They are the "fine" movement controllers.

Let's go through an example of how someone can develop a back problem over time without having any one specific event happen. This is one of the most common presentations of back pain nowadays due to the increased workload people have in front of computers and spending a great deal of time in stationary positions.

Take for instance Alex. He is a middle aged man working a job 5 days per week, 40 hours a week. He was athletic through high school and always tried to stay in shape. He was never very flexible and could not touch his toes, "ever!"

Since college he has worked this same job each week, everyday without fail. It has been about 15 years. He sits nearly all day in front of the computer with moments where he gets up for a meeting here and there (where he is also sitting). He has gained some weight since the athletic years and is not nearly as active in his spare time because he has two kids involved in sports and he and his wife are constantly running them around town and grabbing a bite to eat wherever is most convenient.

He develops a pain that begins in the lower back and really is across a belt line. It is hard to stand straight up after sitting in the chair for a few hours. He ignores it, takes a few Advil and goes on with the day. It will be better in a few days he tells himself.

A few days go by and now the pain is located in the buttock area and it feels like he is sitting on something. He also notices that it has been more painful on the one side of the back to bend down and put socks and shoes on. Still, life is too busy to deal with this.

Now a few weeks tick by and this pain is now down in the back of the leg and thigh and it has become very uncomfortable to sit and drive. Bending forward is getting harder and he has to stand at the kids soccer game because sitting in the bleachers is too painful. After this he has had enough and decides it's time to see the doctor, for it's been 3-4 months of this. The pain at this point is severe in the leg and the doctor orders an MRI.

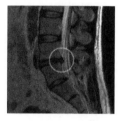

Figure: This is an MRI showing what a L4-5 Disc Herniation looks like. Notice the circled image sticking out of the back

Come to find Alex has one of the most common injuries in the lower back. He has a herniated disc at the L4-5 level. That is what is creating the pain down the leg. So now we have got to the diagnosis, but how did this happen?

Over the years Alex has been in a sitting position 8 hours a day, 5 days per week and for 15 years! That is a total time of sitting of 2,080 hours per year and 31,200 hours in 15 years. Wow! Think about the amount of adaptation that occurred from the cumulative build of sitting all that time over the years. And this is not even taking into account the amount of sitting time driving to work, eating, watching TV, reading, socializing, etc.

So as a result of this, the muscle groups on the front of the legs have shortened across the front of the hip. The muscles down the back of the leg have shortened across the back of the knee due to the joints being in a bent position. This results in more pressure put on the back from the connection these muscle groups have with the bones of the back. The sitting position also forces the discs within the back to be pushed backward. A constant flexed position forward during sitting forces these tissues to "creep" over time toward the back and put pressure on the nerves. Once pressure is put on the nerves, pain will travel down the leg. This often becomes the classic sciatica symptoms so many people are familiar with.

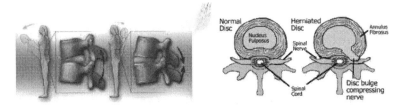

Figure: The picture on the left shows the bending forward of the spine pushing the disc backward. The picture on the right shows how the material of a disc can push backwards onto a nerve.

In the example just covered, the issue with the onset of the pain was never from one specific event. It was the cumulated forces put on the back over time that produced the pain. This makes it so important for people to be aware of the habits, postures, positions they put themselves in over time. Ultimately we may not be able to choose whether or not we can stand or sit for our job. The thing we can control is what we do outside of our job to help offset these forces and keep the body in balance.

Physics Class

I can sense the collective sighs of disgust as I write the title to this sub-heading in the chapter. I realize I am bringing back horrific memories of tedious calculations and theories of things we all sat through in school that had no bearing on our lives, right? Well, maybe? At the most elementary level the human body is millions upon millions of tiny particles moving in space at given rates. Now these particles are always going to do something. They can never remain still. Remember the theory energy can neither be created nor destroyed, just transferred. We are either getting better or worse. We are always moving in some capacity even when we think we are still. So the body is always changing. It will change for the better, or worse. It will change on it's own schedule, or the one you put it on. It's really your choice. So it needs to be mentioned that we control our bodies to a degree. We control what we put in the body to feed/fuel ourselves, we control if we exercise or not, we control if we sit up straight, etc.

The act of what I do everyday as a Physical Therapist is control the way people are using their bodies for the gainful purpose of making the particles do what we ask over time to create a better structure on the inside. Easy? Not quite. When you are dealing with people who have emotions and deadlines to meet, and families to take care of, it can be easy to bypass how you should move and create internal change. After all, internal changes may happen so subtly that you never perceive anything. But if we really break it down, progress is made on the cellular level.

The example mentioned previously talked about how sitting for 31,200 hours over 15 years can create unwelcome change in the body. That is a lot of time devoted to degeneration of the body in one specific position. Now how much time is devoted to working on the body in the manner that would force it to rebuild and get stronger and more resilient to breakdown? Maybe you exercise for 30 min 3 days a week. Okay, so that would be about 1,170 hours over 15 years. Not exactly an equal share of time is it. Now it would be completely ludicrous for me to state we should strike a 100% balance of building activities compared to degeneration to remain healthy. Not gonna happen. I simply present the argument as a logical way to become acutely aware of the time differential spent on different body positions and mechanical strain.

I treat people everyday who are making the choice to improve the health of their back by using movement as their treatment. This is in stark contrast to what the media commercials would like us to think about how just taking Advil morning and night is somehow going to make our back better and more structurally sound and more capable.

No, it will not.

It will pacify the pain being felt by numbing the signal the back is sending to the brain saying , "Hey buddy this structure in your back is in bad shape and you should do something about it before I shut you down."

The vast majority of people out there are just medicating their symptoms. And they will live a life of being the "effect" of their pain. Attempting to find the "cause" of the pain will not be the priority. They will constantly be trying to find the next best mattress, the next best chair, the next best pair of shoes and orthotics to help the back pain. They will never take the bull by the horns and be the "cause" of their improvement. By reading this book and taking the steps needed to slowly change the way the internal structure of your back operates, supports you, and sustains you, you will always be "in control." That is a good place to be.

Pain Is a Response

Everyone hates to be in pain, right? It slows you down, makes you tired, irritable, makes you change your day to day activities and more. All of this is true, however we should all be thankful for the feeling of pain. Follow me for a moment. Have you ever heard of the term Leprosy? This is a real condition and it is characterized by the fact that people who have this disorder can not sense pain! Now you may think this would be great if you were suffering from constant, chronic, gnawing back pain but it could not be further from the truth.

What if you placed your hand on a hot oven and your body did not let you know this was a very bad stimulus and pull your arm back at lightning fast speed. You would be burnt, and badly! The sense of pain is a feedback response. It is not a bad thing at all. It is a signal. Now let's go one step further in the discussion of pain. When the body senses something painful, it is initially nothing more than an electrical signal sent up to the brain. Once the signal hits the level of the brain, it is the brain that will perceive it as pain. I say the word perception because we all perceive pain differently.

I use something called the numeric pain rating scale in my practice. Everyone hates this scale. This is a scale where I ask someone on a scale of 0-10, how would you rate your pain? No pain at all would equal a 0, and pain that is so bad you must go to the hospital is a 10. And the most common response I get right away is, "Well I have a high pain tolerance, so I hate this scale." People will say this because they automatically feel that you are comparing their pain to the person right next to them and there is no way their pain is the same as *mine*. My answer to that is you are right! No one "perceives" pain in quite the same way. This is why one athlete may sprain an ankle and get right back in the game, and another person with the same exact injury and the same exact extent of the injury is completely shut down and ineffective because they hurt so bad. It is the perception that determines the extent of the pain response. The same signal is sent up to the brain, it is then up to the brain to perceive it and determine it as a painful stimuli.

I was at a course not too long along where the speaker was talking about this issue. He described a situation where someone is in the middle of the street and sprains an ankle. As the ankle sprains, it sends a signal to the brain that it is painful. The person feels that there is no way they can get up and walk. Next thing you know, he looks up and sees a truck heading right for him. Right away he is able to jump up and run off the road and out of the way. How does this happen? Well, the brain decided there was a much more important stimulus to attend to than the ankle at that moment in time. Because the brain made the decision it was more important to get off the road then perceive the ankle pain, the ankle did not hurt one bit and they were able to run off the road. The minute they reached the side of the road and were safe, they could barely walk!

This could also be considered what is known as "fight or flight" in the body. We have all heard of situations where a mother lifts a heavy object off of the trapped child, where she never would have been able to do that otherwise. Another example would be the person trapped in a wilderness environment and they must endure harsh conditions for survival. In the moment the perception of what is possible goes away and only action occurs. There is a disregard for what is acceptable under normal circumstances. The reaction I am trying to convey in the body is one of perception relative to the situation. These perceptions are influenced by the subconscious thoughts of the mind, the experiences that shape ones life and so on. Take someone who was chronically abused early in childhood. Their perception of pain is going to be very different from the person who never dealt with injury and got hurt for the first time last week. One person is chronically conditioned to shut pain out mentally, whereas the other person has never known what true pain was.

Let's look at an example of lower back pain and sciatica down the leg. We can have two different people and the same mechanism of injury. The mechanism of injury is a herniated disc that puts pressure on a nerve in the back that causes the pain down the leg. They both have an L4-5 nerve root impingement.

The pressure on the nerve causes a signal to be sent to the brain that perceives pain in a certain distribution down the leg. This is a referred pain. Pain is referred when the cause of the pain is in one location and the pain is actually "felt" in another.

They both have strength loss in the leg from the impinged nerve. One has terrible pain, and the other does not. When a nerve is impinged there can be pain, strength loss, or both at the same time. Strength loss is a motor control issue in the body and would not necessarily have an impact on the perception of pain.

Now given the identical presentations of injury, why can one person be able to function with just strength loss, and the other person be nearly incapacitated from strength loss AND pain? It is due to the perception of pain. For what ever reason the person who felt more pain somehow had a different reaction in the brain than the other person.

This can also effect how well someone would respond to treatment. If a person has a low *perception* of pain, and a relatively positive disposition on their ability to change pain, I will guarantee you every time that person will get better. They will do so with less medicine, and much faster with conservative care. A person who is scared of pain will have to face those fears and overcome them to get better. The perception really does become the reality. It remains one of the most challenging barriers to success in clinical practice.

CHAPTER 2 KEY POINTS

- There are 3 main sections of the spine
- Breakdown occurs over time
- Pain is an indicator
- Pain is not the same for everyone, even if coming from the same spot

Chapter Three

Fear and Worries

Have you ever heard the phrase, "It's all in their head" when someone is trying to explain someone else's pain or problem? I have. I have had other medical professionals describe a patient to me in this way numerous times. The funny thing about it is, this thinking can be totally true!

I am going to cover the psychology of back pain in this chapter. Now I am hopeful that I have not offended anyone with my opening phrase. I mean no disrespect and I am not attempting to alienate someone who has been told this and are very offended by it. I am simply making a point that pain is psychological as well as physical and has been researched many times over in the physical therapy and medical literature.

There are tools out there to measure someones ability to recover, and recover quickly that are totally based on fear avoidance beliefs regarding pain in the back.

You can ask a group of 100 people what area of their body they are most afraid of injuring and I will bet you 9 times out of 10 people are going to pick the back as their number one most feared area to injure on the body. We do not become afraid of hurting our knee the same way we become afraid of hurting our back. An injury to the elbow does not seem to worry us like a back injury. For some reason we simply associate back injury with disability, loss of function, and poor quality of life. We have visions of someone with severe curvature, hunched over, stuck in a wheelchair unable to walk upright. I have treated thousands of people with back injuries at this point in my career and I will say without a doubt, the back worries people, period.

Why are we afraid?

Well, we are afraid of the things we can not see, feel, touch, understand, etc. They are a mystery. Have you spent years of your life studying the back? Do you know the exact way everything in the back interacts and produces pain? I would not expect you to.

Fear and worry occur when things are unknown to us. We tend to dwell on the things we do not understand and scare us. Remember the phrase " The only thing to fear is fear itself." This was from a famous president. That means that *fear* for most people is crippling, even if the reality of the situation is not all that bad.

Take for instance someone looking to start a business. I read a lot of business books and a common theme mentioned is the fear involved for someone going out on a limb to start their own business. It is a scary proposition to do something different, new, and something you do not have all the answers to.

Will I fail?

Will I go broke?

These are fearful questions that are usually on the minds of most when entering the world of business on their own. Now let's go back to using back pain as an example. I remember when I was first going through my own back injury.

"The biggest problem I had to overcome was being afraid of making the problem worse and not knowing what to do to make things better."

I was living every day in constant fear of my condition. THAT was crippling. I was changing all of the activities of the day just to handle my pain. I was spending all my time changing life to handle my pain. I was not attacking it to eliminate it. I was finding ways to cope with it so it could set up shop, get comfortable, and stick around for a while. While that could have been the approach I accepted, I decided it was not for me. I had to develop a better understanding of what was going on to achieve less fear about the situation.

Learning, Accountability, Control

These three words will help to bring you out of the world of fear. These words form a concept that plays on one another. When we know very little about a subject, we tend to be slightly fearful.

If you do not know how deep the water is, do you want to just jump in?

You probably are wondering what lies below. It someone yells "it's 20 feet deep," all of a sudden you have no hesitation to jump in, matter of fact you swan dive in and feel good about it. The decrease in fear is a direct result of increased *learning* about the situation. That increased knowledge made you feel in *control* and you dove right in.

The ability to be in *control* is a big factor. We all like to be in control. When you assume control of a situation, you have a better ability to effect the outcome. So YOU are the cause of your own fortune, or misfortune. You have the ability to get up in the morning and go for a walk or not. YOU have the ability to seek out more information on a given subject and become more knowledgable about a situation, or not. Being in control is a good thing. It allows you to feel at peace knowing you can influence your surroundings.

Being *accountable* simply means staying true to yourself and not giving up. You show up everyday and complete a task for the purpose of reaching a goal. If you constantly make up excuses for not doing something, you assume less responsibility for the situation and lose accountability to yourself. When you plug away, even in the face of uncertainty and not knowing your ultimate outcome, you prove to your own brain and the forces at be that you have what it takes to get better.

Now to put this all together for the issues of pain, fear and worries. *"Fear, worry, and pain all go together."* They influence chronic pain, and they change the daily activities people are willing to do. The more pain there is, the more fear and worry there is. The more fear and worry there is, the more pain is in control.

Here is an example of how someone can break free and take control of their symptoms. You have someone who says "I am in pain and I need guidance." "I need help to break free from the routine of pain."

There are two options someone can use to gain the knowledge needed to become less fearful and take control:

1. You can call Dr. Google and get advice from one million different blogs and become more confused than when you started ......OR
2. You can seek advice from the experts.

A well trained Physical Therapist is your expert for treatment of back pain. Dr. Google can be dangerous. The main problem with google is trying to filter out the good from the bad. It can create paralysis by analysis. This would take you right back to being fearful instead of helpful if not careful.

If you go out to a restaurant and the menu has 100 items to choose from, do you feel a little overwhelmed? Go down the street and look at the menu of a specialized diner and you will find 3 options. All of a sudden you would feel a lot more empowered in your decision because you know darn well you don't want the first two options, so I'll take the other! So choosing to be focused in where you get your information from is very important.

Using the help of a professional can cut down the guesswork of having to sift through the garbage to figure out what is good.

When you receive expert guidance you are immediately increasing what you know about your condition. And we know the more your learn, the less fearful you are. **How often have you heard someone say "I probably don't need the MRI, but I just need it for peace of mind, I just need to <u>know</u> there is nothing bad in there."**

It is strange how people all of a sudden start feeling better once the fear of knowing a grapefruit size tumor is not the cause of your pain!

SO as soon as you start to learn more about your back pain, the more in control you can be. You can now learn how different exercises can take away your pain. If you do certain exercises you can feel better. If you do nothing, you feel worse. Easy, right? Once you are in control of your symptoms with a series of exercises that take pain away when you do them, you can function with less fear, and not avoid certain activities because you are afraid of pain.

Figuring out how to control my symptoms with a series of exercises was the single most important step I took to get better. Before I gained this control, I struggled greatly each day not knowing how severe my problem was, and what I could do to help it. I was helpless to the pain. If the stars lined up I was OK, but I could not control those stars. And believe me I wanted to line them up everyday. As soon as I began to figure out what worked to decrease symptoms my world changed.

I began repeating the same exercise sequence day after day after day. I was a machine.

I enjoyed putting in the effort as well because I saw improvement everyday. Instead of it being work, it became invigorating. I actually became excited about beating the symptoms. None of this would have started however without increasing my knowledge of what was wrong by learning what to do, staying accountable to my own improvement and controlling what I did and when I did it. Yes, it took some discipline.

If you have no discipline, good luck going under the knife. I hope the pain goes away. Just remember once you allow someone else to effect your outcome you lose control, you lose knowledge and you take no responsibility for the outcome. Very different approach from taking control, learning, and assuming responsibility.

CHAPTER 3 KEY POINTS

- Fear can limit your recovery
- You have to learn to take control
- Stop being a "what if" negative person and like Nike says...."just do it!"

Chapter Four

The Usual Suspects;
The Path Most Follow

The path I am referring to here is the traditional way that most Americans seek medical advice for the treatment of pain. Let's say you are sitting at home reading this book and you are in pain. If you think your pain is severe enough to seek care, there are a few questions to ask.

Where do you go?

Who is the very first person you think about calling?

If you are like most people, you have been programmed throughout life from your parents and generations before to be calling a primary care physician. This can also be known as a family physician or an internist. Slight differences, however many people view them the same in the non-medical world.

The primary care physician is known as the gatekeeper. This means they route a person where they need to go. So if someone comes into the office with a cold or flu, they are in the right place. If you come in with back pain, this can be a little more tricky. The typical primary care physician is going to treat back pain in a few different ways.

They may order an X-Ray.

They may prescribe medicine for the pain.

They may prescribe rest as a means to decrease pain.

While these are all approaches that have been around forever, just like a lot of other things in life, we now know better and we have better alternatives that help someone get better faster.

Back pain is not all created equal. If someone has back pain beyond the scope of the primary care they will generally refer them to the next most qualified practitioner. This tends to be an orthopedist or a neurosurgeon. Those doctors are more specialized in the treatment of the back, some will have even completed fellowships in only back surgery. These doctors can evaluate the severity of the condition and make recommendations such as medicine, further imaging such as an MRI, and determine if an invasive approach to treatment such as surgery is applicable.

Now keep in mind, surgeons are trained in surgery. Not every surgeon out there is quick to recommend the knife, however I have seen many cases where they are. Remember they are in the *business* of surgery. The tools at their disposal for helping decrease pain include medicine and surgery. If surgery is not something you want to have, than you should be careful with whom you ask for advice and realize there are many ways to treat the back.

Chances are if you choose to seek out an expert who has spent many years learning and perfecting minimally invasive spine surgery, then I bet you minimally invasive spine surgery is high on their treatment list. If you happen to be a candidate, whoalla.

Never mind if you *could* get better with a less invasive means such as conservative care.

If that surgeon can not sell someone on the notion of surgery, they are not going to be in business long. I hate to say it, but in the field of healthcare, surgery pays. Let me also take this moment to mention I have had the pleasure to work with countless surgeons who are not quick to the knife and truly have the best interests of their patients at the forefront, so I am by no means trying to generalize to all surgeons here.

I am also not naive, even in the field I practice, we are out to remain in business. In the broad scheme of things however, there is nothing sexy about plain old conservative care that takes work on the part of the person looking to get better. Not to mention the fact it is significantly cheaper to complete a normal round of conservative care by a long shot compared to other modes of treatment.

As we get further into this chapter it may seem to some like I am bashing the medical forms of treatment, especially surgery. Realize I am a physical therapist, and I believe in conservative care and allowing the body to be the natural marvel it is.

I believe that conservative care such as physical therapy needs to become even more mainstream than it is and accepted by the public as the authority in the treatment of certain conditions.

With that said the medical model has been around forever, and for a good reason. It has been there is to protect the public from unqualified practitioners missing more severe disease processes that mimic a pain in the back. We call these referred pains.

Just speaking for the Physical Therapy profession, we are trained extensively about screening for "red flag" conditions. We call them "red flags" because they are meant to stop us in our tracks and say, *"Is what we are looking at more than what it seems?"*

If we are evaluating someone with back pain in the clinic and they give a presentation of pain in the back that is unrelenting, does not change with positions, wakes them up at night and has resulted in a sudden loss of weight that they can not explain we need to dig deeper. Physicians are schooled very well in this. They are able to pick this up and perform the correct tests in order to rule out something like the previous stated example which could result in the diagnosis of cancer for someone.

In contemporary Physical Therapy education at the doctoral level (which all entry level practitioners now have coming out of school) there is extensive training on the screening of these conditions which may pop up in your practice and need referred out the door for further testing by another practitioner.

Take another example of someone who suddenly has crushing back pain and they can not move, can not reduce the symptoms, and the acuity never ceases. This could be an emergent condition known as a AAA. This stands for abdominal aortic aneurysm. Something this severe may never even make it to the PT clinic, but if it would, there is no way it should be treated. That person needs the help of a medical doctor immediately.

"Red Flags" are meant to serve as a starter point during a comprehensive review of systems in the body to make sure someone is in the right place and being treated by the right professional. The systems of the body can be broken down to:

- Cardiopulmonary
- Musculoskeletal
- Genitourinary
- Gastrointestinal
- Neuromuscular
- Integumentary
- Endocrine / Metabolic

If a doctor is following the usual medical model, and they have determined a person may be a candidate for conservative care by way of ruling out these more serious types of conditions they may get referred to a Physical Therapist or other healthcare practitioner.

Here is the problem with the tradition method. This process of going to the primary care physician, trying some medicine at first, maybe X-Rays and MRIs, going to the specialists, and making sure all red flags are ruled out can take weeks to months. I will attest to the fact that this is a long time to be in pain. By that point in time conditions generally tend to start effecting other areas of the body as well. Back pain starts to create pain and problems in the hips, which can lead to pain in the knees and so on.

We now have extensive research studies in the physical therapy literature that prove if we can treat someone early we have the ability to decrease pain and reduce the impact of the disability that could result from back pain very quickly.

In a study originally published by a Physical Therapist named John Childs et al they found that by following a certain grouping of findings during a history and exam they could identify patients who would respond to the tune of 50% less pain in 7 days if seen and treated within the first 16 days of pain.

Now to be seen within this window it takes being routed along quickly and to the correct people. This is where the rub lies. The medical community does not necessary know these studies and therefore it's hard to know, what you don't know. People in my profession feel like others should just know what we can do, however there are not enough people out there spreading the word. Medical schools simply have so much to train physicians on, the art of referring to PT is not high on the priority list.

There was a great study conducted and published in the Wall Street Journal a few years back. The authors of the study decided to take the traditional medical model of how people are usually treated for back pain that we had just discussed and they flipped it.

Yes, they treated it 100% in reverse and had people go to the Physical Therapist first and let them determine if they needed further care elsewhere.

Now before you go, wait a minute how are people going to be safer with this method of care by not seeing their doctor first? Let me first say, that today's Physical Therapists with direct access licensure and proper training are every bit as qualified in detecting "red flags" and the need to send patients to more qualified people as needed. If there is suspicion of something more than basic old everyday back pain, you better believe we are getting that person out the door.

As a matter of fact in our own military, Physical Therapists are part of the gatekeeping team. They see patients directly along the same lines as physicians. They can order MRIs, X-Rays, and prescribe basic medication. These privileges are not allowed in general public practice yet, but the training is there none the less.

There are also studies out there that have compared Physical Therapist diagnostic accuracy of muscle and bone conditions that have them ranked higher than primary care physicians, higher than physician assistants and nurse practitioners with only being slightly bettered by orthopedic surgeons.

Now back to the study from the Wall Street Journal. They had found that by seeing a Physical Therapist first, the people got better faster, and it cost less money overall for the person out of pocket. It also cost the healthcare company (insurance companies listen up!) much less when compared to combining all the previous care together by the time someone got to a PT.

You will see in a figure from the mentioned study the significant differences in the costs involved with both models of care. Many people are usually deterred from starting a course of conservative care because of co-pays and feeling that it is more expensive. More often than not when you take away the emotion of having to make consistent co-pays that add up each visit and you compare it to the cost involved with the other options such as surgery or injections, the conservative care is always cheaper.

So I say beware to the person who thinks they are going to "save" money by not committing to taking care of their body with work, sound instruction and doing it a few times a week. The cost is usually less and the overall long term benefit it always worth the effort and time. After all when you are done, not only do you usually have a program to take with you and complete forever, you have gained the knowledge of what to do, the control and power over your pain and condition to fight back on the body rather than just waiting for it to come again and take over your life again.

That same approach to treating the back with a physical means is what this book is all about. It is your way to start a physical therapy treatment method without ever leaving the house!

Throughout this book I am going to be educating you on the process of how pain is treated in our country and how we can look at it differently and come up with better approaches. The process I have just described above of trying conservative care initially for properly screened conditions is gaining traction and becoming more and more popular. In fact in my practice I see a significant proportion of patients directly who have seen first hand these benefits and they are taking charge of their health care.

The 20 minute back solution is rooted in understanding this traditional process and with the correct knowledge taking the bull by the horns and attacking your back condition with physical measures as your first step in the care of your back. This book is not meant to take the place of the knowledge and expertise of your physician or physical therapist. This book is meant to be a guide. A guide that when properly executed, will improve the health of your back now, and in the future. It is about performing a group of exercises in the same manner, consistently, everyday for good.

This solution can work if you are currently in pain, currently just looking to be preventive in nature, or just want to be healthy and well rounded, etc. I am more concerned with the compound effects this solution can have for you long term, over time when completed day after day, month after month, year after year. Small hinges swing big doors some would say. No matter the current state of your back, how many practitioners you have seen for your back YOU can start the journey back to health today. The day you picked up this book was the day you changed your ability to keep arguably the most important part of your bodies structure intact and strong for the rest of your life.

I encourage you to keep reading and take the path less followed and use a very simple formula for the sake of your long term success. In my practice we employ all types of techniques to help improve back pain. These treatments are tailored toward the individual person. For the sake of this book, we can state that this is a general approach for treating the back. It takes the best of each approach and combines it. I made the approach take no longer than 20 minutes because this is what most people who come into the clinic are looking for.

A fast, effective approach they can use within the busy confines of their life. It is the same approach I shared with you in the outset of this book on how I defeated my own back pain.

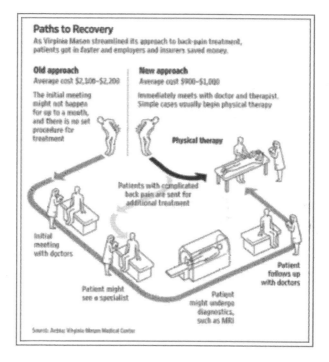

Figure: This is the strategy involved in the process completed by the Virginia Mason Medical System. Published in the Wall Street Journal.

CHAPTER 4 KEY POINTS

🔑 Do you have any red flags?

🔑 For mechanical back pain seeing a Physical Therapist first may be the better option

🔑 The 20 minute solution is THE physical means of treatment to help your back

Chapter Five
Think Like a Mechanic

I like to think of myself as a mechanic of the human body. In my profession, we diagnose and treat mechanical problems in the body. I want you to start thinking about your body in terms of mechanical problems. When you make this type of comparison, it is easier to think in terms of maintenance, alignment, how it runs, tune ups, etc. In the next few sections of this chapter I am going to talk about the body in terms of how we can think about it mechanically. I am comparing the phases of a car's lifespan to the human body in order to make mechanical comparisons.

Nothing Like New

When you go out and buy a new car, everything works. You can drive it fast, not worry about anything breaking right away, and it is functioning at its best. This is pretty much how the body works during youth and the teenage years. You can do about anything you want to it. You can feed it junk, abuse it with ridiculous amounts of sports and high impact activities, and more. Think about the whole entire culture of thrill seekers out there jumping bikes, racing motorcycles, going bungee jumping, you name it. People take their body and the functions it can do for granted when young. Look at the diet of your teenage and twenty some year old kids. Pizza, candy, beer, repeat. They stay up late, sleep in half the day, go run around with friends and do this weekend after weekend.

Remember those days? Yes, you were there too. The body you have today is in part created from the chain reaction of those events over time. Wasn't it nice to just get up out of bed and hit the ground running rather than take the first couple steps out of bed to stand up straight?

I remember the days when I could go to the gym everyday, head out at night on the weekend and not feel a bit of strain or soreness in my body. Then the working world started. Repeating the same actions day after day. Now the main reason the body can withstand all this abuse earlier in life is because of the fantastic ability the body has to regenerate itself even without you doing a thing! It is almost as if the body knows we are to naive and dumb to take care of ourselves so it tries to do it for us. Funny thing is, this doesn't stop! The body is always trying to regenerate itself. This process just needs a little more coaxing along as we age. The repetitive actions we do day after day are what make it hard for the body to keep up the regeneration and it loses the battle. So when the rate of degeneration exceeds the rate of regeneration, the process of breakdown begins.

How to Deal with a Used Car (Used Body!)

So now your body has progressed and you achieved used car status. You are in your late 20s and early 30s. The car is not that bad at this point. But you do need to start paying closer attention to the maintenance of the vehicle to prevent problems. Usually by this point the car needs some new tires, possibly a few other parts depending on how hard you ran it.

Now the body is not in need of replacement parts at this point, but let's say you had an injury such as an ACL tear in high school. Maybe you were part of the crowd who had a car accident in your teen years. By this point in time in the early 30s the effects of arthritis can start to set it. It has been proven that injuries early in life may manifest themselves in early arthritis. No guarantees, but realize it is possible. This is the time in life when we can set up the stage for good health habits and get the ball rolling in the right direction.

Another thing that happens in the late 20s and early 30s is the discs of the back begin to lose water content and slowly become more rigid. This is called the process of degeneration. Yes it begins here. The process of degeneration can take a long time. It is not something that just pops up in a day. Arthritis is one in the same with this. It is during these relatively pain free years that the body begins the breakdown process. The age of 27 seems to be the apex of "generation" in the discs and after that the "de"generation process begins.

Let's say that you get the running bug during this time in your life. This happens to a lot of people who want to find some sort of stress relief from work, kids, etc. They want to bring back the same feeling of athleticism and energy from a few years back, and there are many charitable races out there that people like to be involved with.

Running has a huge following. Now running itself is not a bad form of exercise. I have run two half marathons myself. I like the feeling of the endorphins flowing and getting the heart rate up and breaking a good sweat. One thing that I notice in my clinical practice during this point in life for patients however is that injuries arise from the "weekend warrior" status most people fall into.

What I mean by "weekend warrior" is that most people during this point in their lives are working, maybe raising a family and generally have a lot going on. At this point the cumulative damage of work related activities has started to show up in the body. Let's take for example the computer programmer who sits all day behind the desk. The clock hits 5pm and out the door they go for a good **30** minute run. Oh by the way, they ONLY have time for 30 minutes because they need to be home to cook dinner, get the kids to soccer, and help with homework! Meanwhile the leg muscles are nice and tight from sitting all day, the discs of the back are molded into a flexed position from the sitting position all day, and they want the body to just pop up and get going on that 10 minute mile. What I see as a physical therapist in this situation is tight hamstrings, and abnormally loaded discs in the back creating strain resulting in the process of degeneration. Fast forward about 4 years from this point and that breakdown has resulted in some sciatica due to the fact that the strain which was placed on the disc caused it to fail and the contents of the disc herniated out and put pressure on a nerve in the spine. The person now has pain with driving and sitting at work. Pain moved from their back to down the entire leg. This is how degeneration, and cumulative build of negative forces creates problems over time.

I am sure you can guess what activity is the first thing to stop once the pain is too much; *the running.*

Thinking like a mechanic during this period of time would have a focus on maintaining the flexibility of muscles and joints, thus allowing you to remain capable of completing activities such as running. In this stage of life you want to have the least amount of strain on the musculoskeletal system as possible so that the wear and tear on the body happens at the slowest gradient possible.

Knowing which muscles are the tightest is key to taking care of them. The thing about stretching is that is takes time. If you are already significantly tight, do not expect to become a flexible person just because you start doing some stretching, or join a yoga class. Becoming flexible is about slow progress over time. If you try to make stretching happen too quickly all you do is stimulate the protective mechanisms in the body that prevent tearing of muscles. They will actually fight and work against you if you try to go to fast and too hard with stretching. This is what makes the stretching approach presented in this book so effective. It is meant to take time for a reason. It is to allow the body time to adapt in a positive way, for good!

The Car (Body) Starts Approaching 100,000 miles

So this is not what it used to be with cars. 100,000 miles in todays cars is really not all that much. They still can function quite well if they were well maintained. They may have a few blemishes, bumps, and bruises but you could buy one of these cars and take it another 150,000.

The issue here is that the car just does not look the same. You can see the wear and tear starting to become visible, and compared to a "newer" car it is not as appealing.

Let's call this period of time the 40s, 50s, 60s. Have you heard the saying 50 is the new 40. 60 is the new 50. I have. I treat a great deal of the "boomer" generation. This is the generation of folks primarily in the later 50s and beyond. This age range makes up the vast majority of patients in my clinic. We will talk a little more about the true boomer and senior generation a little later. For now we will keep the 40 year old folks in here as well. In this stage of life we still have quite a bit of ability to regenerate. The problem is that we are programmed into fixed ideas, and preconceived notions of what the body should be at these ages. Most people just chalk up a lot of pain reasoning to "older age." Yes, you will have accumulated degeneration of a certain amount based on how your body was used over the years. That does not mean your body is not capable of changing.

Yes, during the 40s and 50s you are more than likely starting to feel the effects of aging. The aching muscles are real, and the morning doesn't quite feel the same as it used too. At this point the cumulative effects of tight muscles, maybe a lack of strength in key areas show up. The hips may hurt, which in turn changes the dynamics at the knees, which in turn changes the dynamics at the foot and ankle. You get the point.

The body is a wonderful system linking one area to the next. Each is dependent on the other. The cumulative breakdown at one area, leads to breakdown at the next and so on. An interesting fact is that 90% of people over the age of 50 have arthritis when shown up on an X-Ray.

The back in particular will become more degenerated as the discs lose more water content and height. In this phase of life spacing in the body becomes an issue. You could make the argument that the most valuable real estate on the face of the earth is the distance between your vertebrae. If you are not the same height as you used to be there is a good reason for this. If you initially have about 1/4 inch of space between your vertebrae in your 30s due to the height of the disc, and you lose 1/8 of an inch at 8 disc levels in the spine in your 50s, there goes a full inch of height. No one can avoid this.

Once some of this real estate closes down too much there can be issues arise where nerves become pinched and can create pain that travels down the legs. This is a condition known as stenosis and I talk about this a little bit later in chapter 6. There can be fissuring which are cracks on the outside of a disc from repetitive bending forces over the years. There can be varying levels of bulging of the discs or even herniations that arise from change over time and put pressure on some of the nerves exiting the spine. The common thread among this age group that I am trying to get across is that degeneration that **has *been*** occurring over time is now becoming symptomatic.

The Classic Car OR The 300,000 mile Corolla (some cars are better taken care of than others!): Boomers, Seniors

Before becoming offended by this sub-title, read further. This is the time in life when most people are looking to retire, enjoy the life they have created, and be active. The last thing anyone wants to do is to spend the golden years holed up in a wheelchair watching life pass them by.

Watching the life they had dreamed about and spent many years working toward happen without them would be a disaster.

Even worse they could spend all these golden years they worked so hard for just to be put in a home, needing help with even the most basic of tasks of the day. I give the title of being a classic car, or a beat up corolla for a reason. Life is very different for many people at this stage in the game. The car is older and many miles have been logged.

The way I have seen people age in my practice takes on one of two forms:

1. The person who has worked their whole life…hard. They are beat up, and defeated and ready to just let life give them whatever is left. They want to just "hang on."
2. The person who is more vibrant and energetic in retirement than when they worked. There is a general sense of taking care of oneself and they are excited for what it next!

Some people will remain very active, vibrant, and "almost new." I say *almost new* because the ability to function at a high level may come at the cost of a joint replacement. In this phase the body actually does take on the feel of a car. You can get replacement parts! There are limits however.

There are no replacement parts for the back. There are surgical procedures available that create an artificial disc, however these are not performed with nearly the frequency of the joint replacement to the knee or hip. People in the classic car category are ones who are actively taking an interest in working on their health. Classic cars are usually well cared for. For some this is the first time in their life they are trying to do this. They were working, raising a family, and generally too busy during their previous years to exercise regularly, so now they are trying to make up for lost ground. They want to make sure that they use this time to make the rest of life go as long as possible, as independent as possible. Some people like to travel and work to stay in shape in order to do that. Some want to be active with grandkids and they stay in shape for that. The reasons are different but the main point is there is something worth preserving in life, and they are rehabbing their physical health to run the car like it used to.

The other form of person I see are the folks who take on the persona of the used 300,000 mile corolla. If you have a corolla, do not be offended, they are dependable cars! These people have worked all their life, things are breaking down, and they are just trying to hold on and get by. They are generally not interested that much in trying to physically rehab the structure and make it look and run better. They are looking to duct tape certain issues so that they can live to fight another day. This is the example of someone popping pills to numb the pain and keep moving to the next day.

They live a life of anxiety wondering from one day to the next if the car will break down for good. Their health is overall not good. Many medicines are simply "propping" up the bodies natural functions. The hoses (blood vessels) are narrowing and fluids are not moving in the same manner. The body is tight in certain positions and really because there is no "want" to change, the breakdown continues in whatever manner mother nature wants to have happen.

The car is not reliable to travel any given distances for the fear of breakdown, and due to the lack of use it just keeps rusting out and parts keep getting more brittle. One day you go to open the car door to go for a drive and off breaks the door!

Ut Oh. Now what. Then the wheels fall off. Now what do you do. Well, you get hooked up to the tow truck, towed to the junk yard and left to sit.

Sounds kinda like a really bad way to think about the body breaking down to the point where you can not "go for a drive" and having to be taken to a nursing home to sit. Hate to put it out there this way, but it is reality and we need to face the issues at hand if we want to address them. These issues in life never become better if we never face them head on and beat them to the punch. At this point in life people have to choose which type of vehicle they wish to be. Restored and vibrant, or towed away.

The Amazing Human Body

The wonderful thing about the human body is that it has the ability to be influenced and do what we tell it to do. The mind is really the engine that moves the body. Have you ever heard the saying "Mens Sana in courpre sano." This means "a sound mind in a sound body." The mind and body work together. So as we choose to take care of our body this means we are helping both our physical and mental health.

In this chapter we have talked about how to *think* like a mechanic in terms of keeping the body well maintained and working properly over the long haul. It is amazing how well a body can continue to move so long as we move it in a way that keeps orthopedic concerns in the forefront

This means taking a hard look at where you are in the spectrum of life, and begin to address your "maintenance" through exercise. The next item to address then is the risk and reward of certain exercises. I talk a lot about this to my patients on how to think about taking care of their backs. There are hundreds and thousands of exercises out there and not all are good in all situations, however they can all be good in some way.

So what do you do?

Well sometimes it is a good idea to get the help of a professional to get you on the right path. Any good Physical Therapist should be able to help identify the appropriate areas to work on, discuss risk and reward in terms of certain exercises and help to set you up for success.

Nothing against the fitness training industry, but linking orthopedic concerns and fitness takes a deeper look than just the muscles on the surface. Fitness trainers are not trained in this capacity. It takes an in depth knowledge of the internal workings of degeneration, biomechanics, pathology, and progression of issues over time to determine what is good to do long term and what is not.

So your options are to start where you stand and get changing the body or get expert consultation. Would you tackle all the issues in your car yourself? I certainly could not. I would not know where to begin to take the engine apart and diagnose a problem and put it together. If I ever do, please never step foot in the car. It would not make it out of the driveway. The body on the other hand, I can just see it working. It is second nature. I can see the systems working together to produce movement. This is what allows me to make comments about how getting the internal systems working together makes a difference.

The body in its most elementary form is the cells and particles that move to create muscle and bone tissue. They are moving and being influenced by what we put in our body through food, and how we are moving our bodies to force breakdown or rebuild.

I compared the body to the aging of a car in this chapter. The main difference between the car and the body however, is the car will never rejuvenate itself. In contrast the body can be a totally new structure in certain respects about 8 weeks from now when a cycle of physiologic change has occurred. The body is either creating more degeneration or more regeneration depending on what we do. This physiologic change can occur either for good or bad. It will degenerate at whatever rate it wants if you allow it to.

A ship floating in the sea without a captain at the helm is a danger to itself and others to run off course!

You do not want to just let your body drift in the ocean of life doing whatever it wants. Tell the body where to go and be the captain of the ship. Make the back degenerate on your time table. Make it keep building so you keep getting stronger and remain capable of high level activity for many years to come.

The back ends up being a huge benefactor of increased strength and support if you choose to build it for your body. The mind and the muscles can even restore connections from earlier in life to help strengthen and stabilize. The brain is the most magnificent of computers in that it can recall programs from YEARS ago. We need to take advantage of this!

So now that I have compared your body to what type of car you are, let's take a look at the real diagnosis of back pain in the next chapter. These will be the most common causes for back pain in America. I hope it will teach you what these conditions really are and why we do not have to be scared of them.

CHAPTER 5 KEY POINTS

🔑 Think about the body in a mechanical nature

🔑 Breakdown comes in phases and is dependent on the maintenance of the individual

🔑 YOU can control the mechanical breakdown OR rebuild!

Chapter Six

Back Pain Diagnosis 101

I have been talking up to this point in the book about all the reasons to make your body move and why I feel it is most important for you to have a good positive mental attitude toward pain. We have also been talking about being willing to just get the ball rolling and get all the cells moving in your body in a good direction and doing it daily.

This chapter will get a bit more technical and talk more specifically about different back diagnoses that people are going to get from their doctor, and what we are treating in our clinic on a daily basis.

In this day an age we have access to nearly everything at the tips of our fingers. You can find information on anything online. Unfortunately, there is a lot of misinformation on back pain out there in the world, and I love how Dr. Google is always right. I mean everything posted online MUST be correct, right? Buyer beware, not everything you find online is worth it's weight in gold!

So here goes, let's get into the meat and potatoes. Let's talk about the real facts of different types of back pain. If you wish to learn about each diagnosis, great read on. If you want to skip ahead to the diagnosis that pertains the most to you, go right ahead. Remember, this is the kind of book you will refer back to 5-10 years from now when your back pain will be different than it is today.

Arthritis

I have a great deal of patients who refer to Arthirits as their long lost second uncle "Arthur." Arthritis comes to us all at some point and in some capacity. If we break down the definition of arthritis it simply means "joint inflammation." "Arthr" stands for the joint and "itis" stands for inflammation.

This is a book about the back and we will talk heavily about how arthritis effects the back, but realize that it can effect any joint in the body.

The spine has 24 main vertebrae that move and can be effected by arthritis. We talked about this earlier in the book where the spine is made up of a bone, disc, and then bone. This is known as the vertebral segment. Within the vertebral segment, the disc and the facet joints are the main weight bearing structures. The facet joints are where arthritis can take effect. So to understand how arthritis can be widespread, take the lower back for instance where there are 5 lumbar vertebrae. Because there are 2 facet joints at each level, that means there are 10 potential areas of arthritis in the lower back.

If you have ever had an X-Ray or MRI taken of the back you have probably heard of facet joints. When they become arthritic they can produce a spurring. The other common area of bone spurring is around the rim of the vertebrae.

A quick note about X-Rays and MRIs for the back regarding arthritis. Statistics show that within the normal population of people *without* back pain, 65% of people will have abnormalities on X-Rays or MRIs. That means they will have problems show up on the X-ray or MRI, but have NO pain.

90% of people over the age of 50 are going to have some form of arthritis on X-Ray/ MRI. This is a huge number of people walking around with a bad back on the inside but no pain on the outside. If you go through your whole life never having pain and a reason to have an image taken, chances are you had something going on and never knew about it.

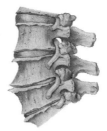

Figure: The above picture is of the lumbar spine showing signs of arthritic spurring.

So with the realization that arthritis within the body can be present in people with or without pain, we have to ask the question, "Why can arthritis be such a source of pain?"

Good Question.

There is a multi-billion dollar industry of pharmaceuticals tailored toward arthritis pain. Tylenol Arthritis (which is really nothing more than a higher dose of acetaminophen with a marketing spin toward arthritis on it), Aleve, Bayer Back and Body, Advil, Motrin.

Ever take any of those? Chances are pretty high you have.

The reason why arthritis effects some and not others is multiple. Arthritis usually becomes painful once the layer of cartilage on the bone called articular cartilage wears away to a layer of bone deeper down. These deeper layers of bone are filled with blood vessels and nerve endings. This is why "bone on bone" can be so painful. Yet there are some people with the bone on bone circumstance, who do not have pain.

This can be attributed to muscular support. The muscles are your shock absorbers. When strong, they can absorb tremendous amounts of force across the surface where the bone bears weight on the next bone. This is how we can "help" arthritis. Most people will always tell me, I have arthritis and I know there is nothing you can do for that.

Well let me be maybe to first to tell you. You are wrong.

There is a great deal of treatment that can be done to help arthritis. Yes, it is true you are not going to rebuild the articular cartilage that has worn away, but your goal changes when you know the layer is gone.

You are then strengthening all the muscles surrounding the joint and keeping the joint flexible to the greatest extent possible. By doing this you can absorb pressure at the joint and ensure it moves as well as it can. This in turn leads to decreased pain.

In the back there are many muscles surrounding all of the joints and bones in the lumbar spine. They connect in multiple criss cross formations in order to turn, side bend, flex, extend, and perform all of the major movements of the body. These muscles are affectionately known as the "core."

"The Core" has become the most popular term in the fitness and rehabilitation industry. Strengthening these muscles is vitally important to the health of the spine. Arthritis is a condition that requires flexibility and strength. If you can adequately support the bones and have enough flexibility in the major joints such as the spine, hips, and knees, then the amount of strain on those areas plummets and pain will go down. The wear and tear on these areas goes down as well.

Degeneration

Degeneration is very common with arthritis. Arthritis in some respects *IS* degeneration. With that said, you can have arthritis and not have any loss of height of the discs, which is typical when the back is degenerated. In order to understand whether the back is degenerated or not, let's consider degeneration to be the breakdown of the disc in the back.

The discs in the back are a form of shock absorption. They are the structure that is between the bones. As the disc degenerates, we lose height and the shock absorbers in the back get more rigid, causing the back to be perceived as "more stiff."

The disc is made up of a fibrocartilage outer ring and a more fluid based material on the inside. The material on the outside of the disc is a tough material. The material on the inside of the disc is fluid, meaning it can move and take shape. It is not a true liquid such as water, but a thicker consistency. Many have tried to explain it as a toothpaste like consistency. It is the material on the inside of the disc that helps to cushion and help the spine bend. It is also the material that protrudes out of the disc if the outer band tears, creating a herniation (i.e. herniated disc).

Over time and many years of use the discs in the body slowly lose water content and become more rigid. As they become more solid, it changes the back's ability to bend, and absorb shock. Sometimes the discs will even crack, which is known as fissuring, and lead to the inside material of the disc leaking out. Again can create herniations.

Many of us out there are not the same height as we used to be. The over 50 crowd is nodding there heads in agreement as they read this statement. If you are not there yet, don't worry, you'll get there too. To some extent we can not prevent mother nature from a natural breakdown of structures in the body. Even if you do everything right to take care of your body you are going to get some form of degeneration and solidifying of the disc. It is what your activities are like day to day that either makes this happen sooner rather than later. The longer the body has to adapt to the change, the better the bodies ability to handle the change without causing pain.

The problem with degeneration is that it is not reversible. You can not add height back to the disc in the spine once it has been lost. This is why it is vitally important to start NOW limiting the wear and tear on these structures in the back so that they move freely.

Degeneration is treatable by making the structures around the joints, as well as the joints themselves as flexible as possible. This is why a stretching routine like the sequence presented in this book is so effective. There is also some evidence out there that loading the spine during a squatting exercise where weight is placed on the back can help to maintain the height of the disc. That is beyond the scope of this book, however an interesting fact to note.

Disc Herniations

This diagnosis is a natural transition from the previously mentioned disc degeneration. A disc herniation can happen as a result of degeneration, but it can also be from a traumatic overload or from repetitive damage over time. This is the diagnosis that is near and dear to my heart due to having lived through it.

As you may have realized from reading my story earlier in this book, I was quite young when I herniated these discs in my back (late teens, early 20s). I was ending my first year of college. So this type of injury is not just for someone who is in there 20s, 30, 40s or 50s. It can effect all groups. As a matter of fact, there are more people in their 30s and early 40s who have disc herniations than any other group. The reason for this is that it is during the 30s and early 40s when the disc still has the capability to "squirt out" some of the inner fluid material and touch a nerve. And these are also active years.

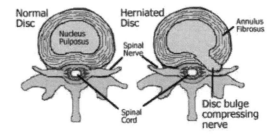

Figure: This illustration shows a normal disc on the left, and a disc with the inner material called the nucleus pulposus on the right extruding out of the outer ring of the disc and pushing on the nerve. This would create a pain down the leg of the person dealing with this injury.

The outer ring of the disc is a piece of fibrocartilage called the annulus fibrosis. The inner more jelly type material is called the nucleus pulposus. The way to think about a herniated disc injury is as follows.

Consider a jelly filled donut. It has the jelly on the inside and a outer layer of dough. If you were to forcefully squeeze down on one side of the donut, you would more than likely "squirt" the jelly out of the other side. The disc will do the same thing if there is too much force during an activity such as repetitive bending forward or sitting for a period of time. The force can come all at once, such as if someone where to jump out of a window, slam the ground and have the trunk forcefully bent forward, or it could come from the vibration of a car or truck seat while sitting in a flexed position over time that pushes the material out.

A person who drives tractor trailer for a living has some of the highest risk for herniated disc injury. The field of nursing has the second most highest incidence of back injury of this kind. The injury occurs because of a failure of the fibrocartilage ring to keep the material inside. Sometimes the fibrocartilage outer ring can also push on the nerve. No matter what, it is this pressure on the nerve that becomes the problem and creates the pain.

There are a number of different words used in the medical world to describe a herniated disc:

1. Disc Herniation
2. Disc Rupture
3. Disc Extrusion

It should be noted, that a disc herniation is the more severe cousin to the "disc bulge." I notice a lot of folks get confused between the two of these. You can have a disc bulge and it pose no significant problem. As a matter of fact, it would be extremely difficult to go through life and not have one single disc bulge. I simply bring this up so that we do not confuse the two. One can be very painful and the other go undetected forever.

A herniated disc usually presents its pain by starting near the buttock and traveling down the leg. Usually it is down one leg only, however there are special cases where both could have involvement. The pain may create a numbness or tingling down the leg. It may also create a weakness in certain leg muscles that correspond with the nerve that is pinched in the back.

In my particular case I had described earlier in this book I had a weakness in the L4 and L5 areas. This made it difficult for me to lift my foot due to these muscles not getting their signal from the pinched L4/L5 nerve. Functional characteristics of a disc herniation will be trouble with bending, sitting, driving, and at times sleeping as well.

Something that is important to note is that there is a very specific type of exercise that benefits disc herniations usually. These have become popularly known as "McKenzie" exercises due to being made popular by Robin McKenzie. This is simply a form of extension of the spine to move the contents of the disc back to a more neutral position and do what is called "centralize" the symptoms out of the leg and into the back.

There is proportion of the population that responds very well to these exercises. Others may not do as well. It is important to be fully evaluated by a professional before just diving into some of these specific exercises.

Sacroiliac Dysfunction

This injury is typically occurring in more active people and can happen anywhere, anytime, to anyone. I say this because usually the mechanism of onset is from some form of activity that involves some bending and twisting or going to end ranges of movement.

The area that pain would be present in is typically on the back of the hip and possibly down the leg. A lot of times a person will grab the small of their back on one side to signify the painful area. This is the area known as the Sacroiliac Joint. The sacroiliac joint, or "SI Joint" is where the spine meets the pelvis. This area can be prone to rotational forces. There is a lot of debate in the Physical Therapy field as to exactly how much movement there really is at this joint.

An injury to the sacroiliac joint can effect someone not only at the area involved, but it can also create symptoms elsewhere by disrupting the biomechanics of the leg at the knee, foot and ankle. One of the biggest problems I see with this injury is that people can let it go and "get by" for quite some time. The joint may rotate out of proper position and someone uses medicine to cope for a while along with basic activity avoidance. This can lead to problems in the other areas down the road.

Since the joint just does not just go back into proper position, a person may operate on a bad joint for quite some time. It is not until the pelvis is put back into the proper position that the person is able to fully become pain free. The usual course for this person ends up being "on again, off again" flares of pain over the months or years.

The good news is that this condition is a very treatable injury and responds favorably to manual therapy techniques such as manipulation and targeted stretching. The routine outlined in this book would be a great way to keep the SI Joint healthy, mobile, and stable. If you have a joint to far out however, manual hands on therapy may be needed.

Stenosis

Stenosis in the lumbar spine is characterized by the progressive narrowing of the spacing called the foramina. The foramina is a hole on each side of the spine where the nerves exit from the vertebrae and go down the leg.

Stenosis by definition is any space narrowing and can happen in arteries, different canals in the body and can happen in any person. By nature it is a progressive, degenerative disease that happens over time. The hallmark person who has stenosis is someone who gets pain in the legs with standing or walking which is relieved with sitting. Someone over the age of 50 is more likely than someone younger to have this condition, although there can be instances of stenosis earlier in life.

This is an extremely common diagnosis in the boomer generation. In most people I am treating in my practice, the main complaint is the lack of ability to keep up with the younger members of their families. They will go on vacation together and stenosis is one of those diagnosis that will cause someone to have to stop and take a break to sit down, wait until symptoms have resolved and then they can continue.

Sound familiar?

It is actually quite embarrassing for someone to continuously be the one holding everyone else back. I have seen people have to completely change their plans due to stenosis. The best treatment ends of being avoidance of painful activities.

One way to tell if you have stenosis is to do a test. If you get pain in your legs with walking around the grocery store, grab a cart and then lean over the bar as you keep walking. If your symptoms decrease or go away there is a high likelihood of you having stenosis. The term used to describe the nerve pain that generates in the legs is called neurogenic claudication. Claudication can also give similar symptoms of a vascular nature where the blood vessels are effected. The main difference is that the legs would not get any relief from bending the spine over with walking if symptoms were coming from a vascular origin.

The main way certain exercise can improve the effects of stenosis is to open up the spaces that the nerves come out from. This is done by maximally flexing open the spine with activities such as bending forward. Sometimes specialized exercises are needed in order to improve the symptoms. There is a number of other effective non-invasive treatments for this condition as well, such as decompression or traction. Both are essentially the same thing. Physical Therapists usually call it traction and Chiropractors call it decompression. This is where someone is laying on a table with a harness around the chest, and a harness around the hips. A machine is then programmed to provide a stretching of the spine to the specifications of the practitioner. It can be a very effective tool for stretching open the spaces of the spine. Manual treatments such as joint mobilization and manipulation are extremely effective treatments as well.

Another form of stenosis worth mentioning here is something called Iatrogenic Stenosis. This is stenosis that is formed post operatively. Many people who have surgery think they are in the clear once they are done, and they do not have to worry about there symptoms anymore. Unfortunately, all too often symptoms return and when this happens it is very likely due to scar tissue build up around the area that was "repaired". This form of stenosis is a bit more difficult to treat solely because it is space occupying. This means that even if you open the foramina as much as possible, it can be difficult to open it fully due to the amount of space the scar tissue eats up.

Sciatica

This is one of the most common diagnosis and quite misunderstood. In all actuality the diagnosis of "Sciatica" is largely a garbage diagnosis meaning any pain that goes down the leg. The problem with this diagnosis is that it is too general. All to often someone with sciatica is treated with the wrong approach for the back and leg pain.

I have heard all too many times about someone trying to do exercises to help their back pain and not getting results or relief of symptoms. If that is the case, then the wrong approach was used. Now if you have sought expert counsel from someone like myself who runs a physical therapy clinic, you probably expect that the person in front of you should know what to do and how to do it. Right?

The fact is that in professional practice you have individual practitioners who have been trained to look and interpret findings in a certain way. This leads to variability in treatment styles. The way they SEE your problem is however they were trained to see it. This is different for all practitioners.

I love the field of physical therapy, but I hate to admit that quite a few of my colleagues are trying to fit square pegs into round holes. They want to fit everyone who comes into their door to the approach they have spent the time and money learning to justify their continuing education courses they so love to take. Some professionals get so caught up in earning a new "certification" we fail to think about if it is the right one.

So the beauty of being someone like myself, I am looking to classify and match the most appropriate treatment approach over ALL the different formulas that are out there. No jamming square pegs into round holes!

Getting the diagnosis of sciatica pinned down to the cause, and then matching the right treatment is the trick for success.

Soooooo, what is Sciatica?

Again, the answer is multiple. It can be from any of the previous diagnoses that we have already covered. Sciatica can come from a *herniated disc* creating pain down the leg. It can come from *stenosis* that pinches the nerves of the spine with standing and walking, creating pain down the legs. *Sacroiliac dysfunction* from a pelvic bone being out of the proper position due to lifting a box wrong that results in pain going down the leg could be a cause. Finally, it could also come from tight muscles called the piriformis muscles which could put pressure on the sciatic nerve. Knowing that sciatica can be any of these conditions is a good starting point to begin an exam because the most important part in helping someone get well is determining what we are treating in the first place!

Scoliosis

I have many patients who come into the office talking about their scoliosis. To clarify, Scoliosis is a abnormal curve of the spine that happens in the thoracic spine, the lumbar spine, or both. It generally curves to the left or the right.

Most of us were exposed to the diagnosis of scoliosis early in life due to the screenings that students will receive going through grade school for various physicals. Have you ever seen the test where the nurse or other healthcare provider is behind the patient and asks them to bend forward? They are looking for something called a "rib hump" that would be protruding on one side of the middle of the back. If this is spotted, the child would then be referred to their doctor for further care. Some adolescents who have scoliosis will simply be treated with observation, strengthening of the muscles surrounding the scoliosis, and stretching of the muscles that would shorten due to the abnormal curve.

In the more severe cases, someone would need to be placed in a brace to prevent the curve from causing further problems. For the scope of this book, we will not cover the details of when one should be braced or whether the scoliosis is fine to treat with basic stretching and strengthening. That should be a decision made by your healthcare provider.

While we usually think of the previously discussed adolescent as having scoliosis, we usually do not necessarily think of scoliosis as a **degenerative condition.**

Think about the way the spine is configured. It is a series of curves. Usually these curves stay in one common plane which is generally called the sagittal plane, meaning it goes straight front to back. It is when the curve goes into the frontal plane, which is side to side that a problem ensues. Now when discs degenerate there are multiple forces placed on them from a number of different directions.

"There is no rule that says discs have to degenerate straight up and down."

One side may break down more than the other and this would cause a wedge looking disc effectively tipping the vertebrae above it on an angle. If this occurs it makes everything up above it go on an angle as well. In order to compensate and get the body level to the horizontal, the body will develop a curving position to accommodate. This will make someone with advanced degenerative disc disease look like they have a curve to the back. This could be evident on X-Ray, as one would be able to see how the degeneration actually looks.

The point I am trying to make regarding scoliosis, is that it can be from a few different cause. Some are more treatable than the others.

The form of scoliosis from degeneration could be amendable to change with conservative treatment. We would not expect the same type of results with fixed scoliosis from one's youth. It is not that we can not do anything for these folks, that would be the furthest thing from the truth, I am simply saying we have more ability to impact the degenerative type of scoliosis with stretching and strengthening.

Instability

The diagnosis of instability is deceiving. I am not referring here to someone who has freely moving bones within the spine that are "unstable" due to a fracture of the spine. I am referring to someone here who lacks the ability to use their own "core" muscles effectively to keep the spine in a neutral position.

Have you ever heard of someone saying they threw their back out trying to pick up a sock?

Yes, a sock!

Why would this happen trying to lift such a light object? The reason is due to a momentary lapse in the neuromuscular control of the spinal joints. Instability!

Another example of instability is the brick layer who lifts and moves heavy blocks all day long. Overall they may have a pretty good muscle build to the naked eye. They come home and bend to pick up a child's toy off the floor. They drop to their knees because the back "goes out". This is a very common diagnosis and one that has to be treated with strengthening of the abdominal and lumbar muscles.

Instability has been described in many research articles, and we know that it can be a difficult diagnosis to treat because it not a fast moving diagnosis. Stability is something that has to be developed over time through the building of muscle. It is always easier in my professional opinion to try and take a stiff, tight structure in the body and loosen it, rather than to try and take a very loose and unstable part of the body and make it tighter.

We make things tighter naturally by using strengthening exercises. It is incredibly popular to talk about "The Core" these days. Many different disciplines from yoga, to Pilates, to various other forms of physical training try to talk about strengthening this region and there are countless ways to do it. I am not going to try and teach you how to perform *all* the different exercises in this book. The more important part is trying to identify whether or not this is the diagnosis that fits you and then tailoring an exercise routine for your needs.

People with instability tend to have certain characteristics. We know based on certain predictor rules that women under 40, who have very good hamstring flexibility, trouble raising their body back up from bending forward (generally termed a thigh climb, where you would walk your body back upright by using your hands rather than the muscles of the back.) , and a positive test called a prone instability test.

No one test in isolation is really good for determining the diagnosis, however this basic grouping of items has shown some promise for identifying people who genuinely need to get stronger and tighter.

Instability can also occur from chronic "adjustments." I see this group often, and on the whole this is the group who has been to the chiropractor off and on for the past 10-20 years. They go in for their monthly "adjustment" or more often depending on the person, get "popped," feel some relief and then the cycle repeats next month.

This ongoing approach to constant loosening is what creates the instability. If all that is ever done to treat the spine is manipulation at the end range of the joint without adequate stabilization around it, one will have this instability type of pain.

I see it nearly everyday.

Now make no mistake about it, I have no problem with manipulation of the spine. I have a practice built around mobilization and manipulation. Most people do not realize that as a physical therapist I do this. We will talk more about this later in the book. The point I am currently getting too is that ***manipulation is shown to provide short term relief of pain, not long term.*** You need something <u>more</u> to influence the body over the long haul.

The long haul solution is strengthening the body to take care of itself. This book is predominantly geared toward a flexibility approach for the sole reason that it is the one thing that can be universal to anyone with back pain. The muscles focused on through these stretching techniques are in all of our bodies, and tend to be points of problems for many people. For further work on the back, getting a proper exam and diagnosis from a movement expert such as a physical therapist is key.

CHAPTER 6 KEY POINTS

 There are many different pain diagnosis

 Sciatica is many things

 Treatment needs to be matched to the symptoms/diagnosis

Chapter Seven
Drugs, Injections, and Surgeries

I once sat in a doctor's office where I had met him for lunch. He was a referring doctor in the area and I wanted to talk to him about the benefits of physical therapy. He told me his thoughts on physical therapy. He thought, **"It was a great way to distract someone's attention from their pain while time helped them get better. We really didn't do anything else."**

Wow, talk about belittling another professional right in front of them.

Fact is, he did not see me as a professional on his level. I was the lowly (however Doctorally educated) Physical Therapist begging for the scraps of his referrals for that week. His opinion was that the only way the back was truly being "treated" was with drugs, injections, and surgeries.

I was not even thought about for legitimately taking pain away as someone who uses stretching, and hands on treatments for relieving pain. Although the meeting bothered me greatly, I can not really blame him alone, it is how he was trained.

He was old school, and not very open to advancements in other professions. He was working from the tools he had learned in the years of medical school and the preconceived notions he had developed in his head about what works and what doesn't.

Let me first start off by repeating that I am a Physical Therapist. I am a practitioner who treats pain with movement: not drugs, injections, or surgery. While I have used medicine personally, had injections to the spine personally, and understand surgery is needed for some, I will tell you there are an equal amount of people out there in pain who do not need these interventions.

In my professional capacity, it is beyond my scope to prescribe medicine, order imaging, or inject the spine. Physical Therapists in the armed forces can do much more than the average as they have limited capability to order imaging and prescribe basic medicine, however this is not practiced in mainstream physical therapy. I have willingly advised patients follow their doctors advice to take medicine, and I have also recommended patients get an injection or visit the spine surgeon when a condition is appropriate for that. What I want you to understand however, is that these are usually the last options I am placing on someone. The main reason for me considering these options after conservative care has a lot to do with the tools each person uses to help someone. Let me explain.

Earlier in the book we talked a little bit about the normal sequence in which most people in pain follow. Pain starts, does not go away, so we see our doctor. Doctor prescribes medicine and rest and orders an X-Ray. Those are his tools. Pain continues, so they go to the specialist. They use their tools. On it goes.

In the world of pain we all have the tools of our trade to treat pain. So depending on who you go to see, there ability to help you relies solely on the tool they can help you with. If our particular "tool" can not help you, than we are obligated to refer you to the next person who can help you. To elaborate further, what I am talking about has a direct impact on what you "think" you need to get better. If you "think" you need a certain treatment, than you have to go to the right person who uses the right tools, make sense? People who see me, who "think" they need surgery, generally do not do as well with conservative care. I do not use the tools of a surgeon.

If you go to the doctor for your back pain and ask for help, how do you think she will help? They will use their tool....**Prescribe medicine.**

This is not rocket science. Medicine is the *tool* of the primary care physician for treating back pain.

Now let's go one practitioner further. A Physiatrist is a pain management and rehabilitation doctor. They are going to perform various tests and the main way they help pain could be with oral medicines or more commonly these days with injections. There are different types of injections out there, but let's not try to get too technical here. I am just trying to explain the tools people are using.

One step further down the chain we have the orthopedic surgeon or neurosurgeon. These professionals are trained in the medical management of the spine and how to perform surgical procedures of the spine. The tools are surgical instruments. So each different doctor has a different tool they use to help your pain.

Now that I have you confused on who you should see for your pain, let's go over a a quick example to help clear the air. If you have a herniated disc you could see a physical therapist OR an orthopedic surgeon. If the disc is a large enough herniation, the surgeon may recommend surgery. The physical therapist may recommend extension exercise of the spine. Who should you believe? Which one of the two will help you the most? Arguably they both have value. This is the reason I am spending time talking about where you go for your advice is for good reason. The tools used between these two professionals are totally different! In a world where each one of these professionals can be an *option* for treatment, you will tend to get the opinion of whatever treatment that person is an expert at dealing with. There has to be an element in there of what YOU want out of the treatment. You will be able to make a better choice the more educated you are. You may not have realized you could be treated without surgery!

I said the word "option" earlier because a lot of spine treatment truly is about options. There is acupuncture out there, massage, dry needling, and they all claim to give more pain relief than the next. Now, if you go to the acupuncturist for pain relief, what do you think they are going to do? If you go to the massage therapist for pain, what do you think they will do? If you go to the pain management doctor for pain and they do injections, what do you think they will do? Get the picture.

Surgery

The mainstream medicine treatments out there are drugs, injections, and surgeries. Would it surprise you to know that the number one determining factor for someone having back surgery is not the extent of their injury, not the diagnosis being treated, but the zip code they live in? I am not trying to offend the back surgeons out there, just educate the lay person on some of the facts.

Certain geographic areas and groupings of surgeons will do more back surgeries than others. Is this solely because they have more people in their area who need surgery? I can not answer that.

Back pain is challenging for the patient to know where to go and who to trust. You would like to trust in the fact that every practitioner you see will be truly looking to treat you in the best way possible and to your values.

Think about the job of a surgeon. If you go see a surgeon and they feel you are a surgical candidate who would do well with a procedure, they are more than likely going to recommend that procedure. Makes sense.

That is their job, that is how they make a living.

Here is where an insulted surgeon is going to lay into me on how they did surgery on someone who would have never recovered without an operation and they are better than ever. To that story I say great! I can talk about a story to match that where it turned out the other way.

This book is not about painting surgery in a bad light, it is on advocating that there are many options out there in the world of treatment for back pain.

Now let's say that this same person who the surgeon recommended surgery for, went to see a Physical Therapist (PT). Would it come as a shock to you that the PT would recommend conservative care? Who is right? Well they both can be to an extent. There are many surgical cases that when treated conservatively in the proper manner improve greatly. Some don't.

Some of what you think may make one right over another may deal with perceived levels of expertise. On the whole surgeons are regarded in a higher light than physical therapists. Despite that fact, just because someone CAN do back surgery and recommends it does not make it the RIGHT choice. In the world we live in, a Physical Therapist's opinion may be weighed with less significance due to perceived levels of training and expertise. We may think advice is right only because a so called expert says it is. It is up to you as a consumer to be educated to the options on the table.

I see way too often someone who is a good candidate for continued conservative treatment give up on it early because their doctor said it'll never work and they are wasting their time they need surgery. And guess what, they call me to cancel all their appointments, thank me for the hard work and tell me "yeah my surgeon said this is not going to work." This is despite improvements in function, less pain and general movement in the right direction. What happened is that they threw in the towel to soon because someone *perceived* as an expert squashed their desire to get better without surgery prematurely.

Maybe the surgeon would be right, or maybe they thought they had a good surgical candidate on their hands. The point here is that the option to get better conservatively was alive and well, but got taken out of the picture for what is thought of as a "quicker fix." In my experience, these quick fixes come with a price, financially as well as physically down the road. People sacrifice long term gain for the "hope" of pain relief NOW.

The surgical push is a play on the psychology of an individual. If someone keeps swimming in the ocean long enough they may wonder if they are going to get to dry land. So the notion of someone coming along in a helicopter picking them up saying you'll never get there without ME is VERY appealing.

Who cares that the helicopter dropped you off an a deserted island with no food or water. They got you out of the water didn't they!

This is all to often the surgical case. They can get you out of the never ending routine of stretching, strengthening, and walking and do a "procedure", but how do you know where you are heading after? The truth is you don't know. So we need to be careful of whom we take directions from and shop around. Get multiple opinions. Talk to people who use different "tools." If everyone is on the same page, then you can proceed with confidence, not based on fears and worries of what will happen without it. Fear is a big motivator of decisions.

Fear is such a big motivator, which is why we covered it earlier in the book. I find that people become consumed in decisions based on what they are afraid of. Many people come into our clinic afraid of doing more harm than good. There is a thought out there that by coming into a place like our physical therapy clinic that we are going to make them worse. Now I will say there are bad apples in all professions but we certainly are not in business to make people worse off. Why are people worried that learning how to move their bodies properly will make them worse? This comes from the fact that they are trying to already move better at home. They have made adjustments to their life to help accommodate their pain, how could you make them move any different?

I am asked..."How do you think moving my body is going to help? Moving hurts me!" They will say, "If I just sit still I'm good." Well if you sit still the T-Rex can't see you and won't eat you so you should never move again. I hate to say it, but if you plan on living on earth and doing anything productive in life, you will have to move. And pain, like the T-Rex, can either eat you alive, or you can learn how to take it down.

The fear people have seems to evaporate somewhat however when in the hands of a trained surgeon. So let's go over an example.

I prescribe someone some basic everyday movement stretches in my clinic like pulling a knee up to the chest. It hurts. That person then thinks you are out to hurt them, does not think you know what you are doing, and then is all too willing to sign up with the next surgeon who they heard was good.

Forget the fact that you met the surgeon for 5 minutes, surgery was decided on, and next thing you know they roll your body into the operating room. You proceed to let this perfectly fine stranger spend the next 4-8 hours cutting you up, screwing, plating, and sewing you back up to have free reign over your body. Talk about trust.

We are willing to do that, but not willing to stick with doing some stretches? There has to be some reasoning for putting this trust in someone to do a massive surgery over some simple stretches. Could it be because you are afraid if you just kept stretching you would get worse?

Now I understand some of you out there are all about staying *out* of surgery and I hear you. Just realize there are a LOT of people out there all to willing to lay on the table without any further regard to their body.

The fear of having such a dramatic surgery can just melt away because of the authority of the surgeon. He or she is highly skilled, spent years training all to protect and help decrease your pain. We see these folks as the authority on what will or will not work for the treatment of the back. I know some surgeons who seem to recommend surgery for all cases they feel meet certain criteria whether or not they are a conservative care candidate. There are other surgeons who will have folks exhaust all options before performing an operation. Good apples, and bad apples. They are everywhere. Undoubtedly I have offended some with my views here. The main point to take home here is that fear is a HUGE factor in how someone will choose to be treated.

On the flip side of this some people may actually strong-arm a surgeon into doing a surgery they really do not want to do. People may try to convince a doctor to prescribe drugs that they really do not think are necessary. We make health decisions based on not wanting to hurt in an emotional state. This obviously is not the best state to make a decision in, and will ultimately effect the outcome on the other side.

Spinal Injections

I have spent some time now talking about the pitfalls of rushing into surgery prematurely. On one hand you have a surgeon who may suggest surgery over conservative care, or you can have someone who actually just pushes for the surgery. Since surgery is not the only option for people let's spend some time talking about another option for those who want to stay off of the surgical table.

I was in this category personally. This is where someone may opt to have injections of the spine. This form of treatment is thrown out there a lot now with varying levels of success. There are a few different types of injections out there. I will not talk about all of them. Injections are not my area of expertise. I can play a role with when to suggest them for someone in need, but I do not give them. A pain management doctor is the expert there. What I will talk about are the two I see most often in my practice. I see people who will get facet injections, and epidural steroid injections.

Facet Injections

These are injections that are administered to the actual spinal joint perceived to be the one creating the pain at the articular surface. This means where the bone meets the bone. This is different than the epidural steroid, which we will talk about in a minute. Facet injections may have a benefit for someone dealing with joint based pain such as arthritis or degeneration which creates a more bone on bone feel. The problem with this is in identifying who should get them or not. I will speak from my professional opinion that I have noticed the improvement in people seems to be no better than the flip of a coin. People who I thought would benefit did not, others did. With some things in healthcare, you simply do not know until you try in terms of pain relief. We are all in the race to prove the worth and effectiveness of our treatments. This one can work for some but not for others.

Epidural Steroid Injections

This is the more common of injections I see clinically and the type I have had personally as well. An epidural steroid injection is placed into the space in the spine known as the "epidural space". This puts the medicine into a very selected area of the spine where it can be right on the level of the nerve that is trapped. Doctors determine the level by taking an MRI of the spine to see where the entrapment occurs. The injection is meant to be anti-inflammatory in nature with some pain relief component as well. The problem with most of these injections is knowing who to give them to, and where in the sequence of treatment. Again, I see the effectiveness being more 50/50. An injection is usually not the first mode of treatment someone is getting for spine or sciatic pain. People are generally referred to one of these doctors after another doctor has determined that oral medicine did not work. These are cases where the person is not meant for surgery (or does not want surgery), and they may or may not have done physical therapy. Sometimes this whole process takes weeks to months.

There are two main downfalls to the epidural injection in my eyes. One is not knowing who should get these and who should not. This has been brought up more recently in different medical journals. The Journal of Family Medicine brought light to the issue that these injections are getting totally overprescribed and used in the absolute wrong cases. This is due to a lack of good criteria for choosing who should get one.

I had these injections done for two reasons.

1. My pain was not going away, and I refused surgery. The surgeon I saw was on board with the injections as well since I was relatively young and healthy otherwise. It was not until I was in pain for a few months however that the injections were even presented as an option. What is most perplexing to me now, is that no one had even mentioned the possibility of doing physical therapy for me despite learning through training that I would have been the ideal candidate. I may have not had to endure such pain if I had been able to give it a try. So getting back to the injection and the fact that we do not know who we should be giving them to, it is hard to recommend the ideal candidate.

2. The second reason was to shrink the disc. Sounds good in theory, but the biggest downfall of the injection is the inability to create true lasting mechanical change. I was told prior to my injections that they "were going to shrink the herniated disc back into where it came from." This sounded great to me. I am still unsure to this day if it really did. I have no repeat MRI to prove this. What I will say is that the injections gave me marginal pain relief to begin the true essence of what I needed to recover, and that was to get moving.

I am sure the injections alone would not have got me to where I ultimately wanted to go. This is the downfall to some people I have seen who get an injection alone. They expect a miracle because they just want relief. Some are vastly disappointed. I find better results from those who are coupling the injections with true mechanical treatments via exercises to build the body back up and improve the structures that ultimately created the herniation or degeneration in the first place.

Oral Medicines

The number one most commonly used treatment form for back pain in our country (USA) is oral drug therapy. I single out the USA because other countries and cultures are not as fast as we are to pop a few pills and keep pushing on through our days.

Turn on the TV at any point in time during the day and you will see a handful of pharmaceutical commercials pitching different drugs. In fact we are so used to seeing such commercials, and so blind to drugs that some of my patients when asked to list the medications they are currently taking in their patient history form, they do not list Ibuprofen, Advil, Aleve, and Tylenol on the list.

When I ask if they have been using any of these they say, "Well yes I have been taking that!" It is almost as if they are so commonplace anymore in our culture that we do not even recognize them as drugs, capable of exerting harmful effects. The fact that you can get them over the counter next to the vitamins makes then "less dangerous" in the minds of the consumer. So in turn, some people think of these as first line defenses. And the companies advertising of these products want you to think that as well.

Take for instance the gentlemen in the Aleve commercial who is a postal carrier and tries to "get through his day without his Aleve." My goodness let's not do that! How could you do such a thing? I NEED my Aleve. If I don't take it, somehow my legs will stop working and I will not be able to walk!

What is the reason most people are taking Aleve? In one word, Pain. The drug has a role in this. The drugs chemical role is to help eliminate the pain. It does this by changing the signal sent from the pain generating part of the body up to the brain so that the brain does not receive the pain signal. It essentially "blocks" the signal.

The medicine will not FIX the mechanical problem.

That is why the fine gentlemen carrying the mail in the commercial will have to take it everyday for the rest of his years until he gets his knees replaced. Or until the back is fused together to limit the ability of the individual levels of the back to cause pain.

So what would happen if this same person decided to strengthen his legs and adequately condition his body to absorb the force at the knees which would STOP the pain all together? *Well it sounds great but does not sell too many pill bottles!* It takes a lot of money to manufacture drugs.

Oral medicines come in many varieties.

You have NSAIDS, which are non-steroidal anti-inflammatory drugs. These are the Advil, Aleve, Motion, Bayer Aspirin class of drugs. They are all trying to perform relatively the same action. NSAIDs will effect a couple different parts of the body when placed into the system however. They will make an attempt to decrease pain, and decrease inflammation, but they are also quite harsh on the lining of the esophagus and the stomach. This has lead to GI bleeds and other complications from the use of NSAIDs.

I do a great deal of joint manipulation/mobilization in my practice. Some people are scared to "have the back cracked," but are all too willing to pop Advil day after day in quantities above the recommended limits. An interesting fact is that it is *safer* to have the spine manipulated than it is to take Advil. More people are hospitalized each year in a landslide from GI bleeds due to NSAID use over people who have an adverse reaction to joint manipulation. Matter of fact, rarely if *ever* is someone hospitalized after joint manipulation.

There are also a class of NSAIDS out there known as Cox-2 inhibitors which include Celebrex as being one of the more popular drugs in recent memory. The action of these drugs is supposed to decrease the risk of stomach irritation by the inhibition selectively of Cox-2. You do not really have to know more of the technical aspect of these drugs for neither you nor I (unless you are a physician) will be prescribing these drugs.

Oral narcotics like Oxycodone, and Vicodin are way too popular, and are beginning to get more regulated as we speak. The action of these drugs is meant to be at the level of the central nervous system. It works to decrease the brain's response to the pain signal being sent up from the source.

This is why people are often sluggish and do not feel "right" when taking these drugs.

It is also why they need to discourage people from operating heavy machinery when taking these drugs. The mental capacity of these folks is altered with slower processing. These are also the drugs that are abused and often sold on the secondary market for there heroin-like properties. It is for these reasons I have a lot of people who do not want to take these for fear of addiction, and some because they want to actually have an awareness of there pain so that they can work on correcting it, not just blunting the pain. This is in contrast to the person with Kidney stones who could benefit from the use of these powerful drugs to dull the pain from a process they can not just go stretch out to get better. So these drugs have a role in medicine, make no mistake about that, just not in the long term treatment of back pain.

Am I Anti-Drugs?

It may seem so at this point.

If you have taken anything away from reading at this point, you know that I have talked extensively about the downfall of treating pain with drugs. To my colleagues out there who will not take kindly to this bashing of drugs, realize I understand they have a place. I am not totally against someone using ibuprofen to reduce their pain, and there are times I will suggest it myself to someone.

"Inflammation is inflammation," and when out of control needs to be calmed down before going into fixing the mechanical problems. I get that. My main focus on the discussion in this chapter is the huge mental fixation we have with drugs "fixing" the issues at hand.

When combined with the proper structure building methods (i.e. stretching and strengthening) the results can be quite good. The problem here is that society just views the drugs as THE treatment. There is no follow up with stretching and strengthening. There is no FIX. It is the fixing of back pain that I am concerned with. My goal remains teaching people how to have a healthier, pain free back naturally. So if you are a physician out there reading this with absolute furious blood boiling resentment, please calm down. I know that YOU know these things. There are many people that do not however.

CHAPTER 7 KEY POINTS

 There are many ways to treat back pain.

 Medicine takes you only so far

 Medicine is more effective for back pain when used WITH the physical treatments

 Is exercise the best medicine?

Chapter Eight

Why Physical Therapy Helps: But Choose Wisely

I have said it before, I am a Physical Therapist (PT). My profession deals with treating pain through the use of the body itself, naturally. Our belief is that the body needs to be treated with a physical means to fix mechanical problems. We are highly trained in exercise techniques and have arguably the highest level of knowledge in this domain of all professions, period. There is no trainer out there that will have the skill set of how the body works and functions through the use of the muscles and bones as a physical therapist. And this is not a knock on trainers. Some are good, but some also just got a mail order certificate stating they can train people. This is not knowledge and skill, but mail order credentials.

Even within the profession of Physical Therapy itself, there is variation in the caliber of physical therapists. This is a function of where they received their training, what they want to specialize in and more.

There is an alphabet soup complex among a lot of PTs out there hungry for letters to put behind there name stating they are "certified" in some technique. In the medical world practitioners love to put a lot of letters behind their name, somehow making them an "expert" at something. In some instances this is no better than the trainers version of a "paid-for" certification. Certifications makes someone want to USE them, and it often results in someone jamming a round peg in a square hole. In some respects these certifications narrow the focus of someone too much, and they miss broader issues. Now I will say this is not everyone, but a good bit.

In our profession we are steadily becoming Doctors of Physical Therapy. In fact there are no longer any lower entry level degrees. Physical Therapists trained a few years back may not have a DPT (Doctor of Physical Therapy Degree) but would have undergone training and past licensure just the same to practice Physical Therapy.

In our field we have residencies and fellowships that culminate in TRUE credentials that take time, study, and board certification. These are the only letters in my mind we should look for beyond traditional PT credentials that will confer to all people graduating from Physical Therapy schooling.

Some schools are better known for orthopedics, neurology and so on. As a consumer looking for the right person to be treated by, this is something you should take the time to be aware of. In the end you can have two people trained exactly the same and produce different results. It's like having two people cook the same thing. They each have their own recipe and without a doubt one is going to taste better than the other. What makes the one taste better? Is is the ingredients used, the way they apply them, and the art of the cooking.

Another example is having two highly skilled surgeons. What makes someone want to seek out and go to the surgeon who may be hours away opposed to someone who should do the same surgery in your hometown? It comes down to how they are perceived, the respected ART of their surgery, the ability to get people better, etc.

The same thing should be happening in the field of physical therapy. It is all to often that the *ART* of the application is what makes the difference. The sad part about PT is that people think of it more as a commodity than anything else. Commodities are things we feel are the same no matter who we get them from, or where we get them from. A common example is oil. Gas is gas, right? We look for the cheapest gas station and go there. With the fact that there are so many places to go for PT and people to see, some feel they should just find the closest person to their house and hope for the best. I hope it works for you.

A lot of people and doctors fall into this trap of all PT is the same. Wrong. Could not be further from the truth. If you truly want to decrease your pain and become well, the right person/place makes all the difference. It also comes down to prescribing the right exercises in the proper sequence as well. Good thing you are going to learn a bonafide stretching approach in this book that the pros use! And all for less than one co-pay!

If we break down the definition of ***Physical Therapy***, it simply means "therapy through a physical means."

If we break down the definition of ***Drug Therapy***, it simply means "therapy through a drug means."

What I want people to think about it is that physical therapy should be considered the all natural physical "drug." We should *"take"* physical therapy to keep our bodies healthy. Physical activity has been shown in countless studies to be the "cure" to diabetes, heart disease, and many other chronic diseases. Now this is a book on back pain in using a physical means to treat the back, however just think for a second about all the other positive benefits of using a physical means of treatment. This is the total opposite of all the side effects of drugs! I should create a commercial on all the benefits of physical therapy as a mode of treatment and then list all the side effects like a traditional drug company would at the end of the commercial. Do you know what it would sound like?

"Using Physical Therapy to treat your back pain may result in more energy, lower blood pressure, less spikes in your blood sugar, decreased pain in OTHER areas of your body from arthritis and more. You were not even looking to decrease your pain these other areas, but it happened. And by the why, you also could have weight loss, better posture, and more. Please let your doctor know about these side effects!"

Wow. If I only knew about something I could take for my pain that would result in those potential "side effects!"

I am trying to make a point with this. You will never see this commercial on TV. It does not have mass appeal believe it or not. We all know that being physically fit is healthier than not being physically fit. We all know that it can have "positive" side effects. Despite this knowledge we continue to rapidly become a nation of increasing obesity and acquired lifestyle diseases. It is the fact that physical therapy takes "TIME" to do that may be the kiss of death. I often think about this time issue. Many times it is the person who constantly says they do not have the time to do these things that eventually ends up not being able to do anything at all because they have retired on some form of bodily disability ready to spend the rest of their life frustrated about what they can no longer do. Once your time is taken away from you, it takes on a different meaning. One that many people if they could have done it in reverse would have invested that small amount of daily time in their bodies for a greater return later in life.

You may be reading this chapter and saying to yourself, "OK, I get this, it all makes sense, but I still do not know <u>where to start.</u>"

If you are saying that, than great. At least you made your mind up that you are ready to take some action and begin the process of using a physical means to build your body so it is more resistant to breakdown, and help it function better for all aspects of your life.

Using a physical means to treat the body is a way to directly attack the negative consequences that occur as a result of natural deficiencies or poor body mechanics. Body mechanics meaning nothing more than how the body moves or sits at rest. Poor body mechanics have a tendency to creep up over time. You may be a naturally tight person regarding flexibility, or on the other hand you may have always been able to touch your toes, bend over backwards and have a relative "gumby" disposition. No matter what the issues are at hand, if they are mechanical in nature, then we have to fix them with a mechanical means.

For example, if a bridge begins to collapse, you can generally see cracks beginning, some pieces may fall off, there is some form of visual damage. One could just try to resurface the bridge. Resurfacing the cracks will make it look better for a period of time. That is one approach. But the issues will be back. Why? It is because the mechanical structure of the bridge was failing and all we did was give it a cosmetic facelift. We did not look to structurally support the areas that caused the cracks. If we had, we would have fixed the problem and not allowed the cracks and situation to return.

Here is where the body is vastly different than other things such as cars and bridges, and other objects. While you can replace the tires on the car, or create a pillar to support a bridge, you have to break the body down in order to create a "rebuild" from within. You do this in order to improve a structure and create change.

What do I mean by breakdown?

The act of working out or completing physical therapy is the process of breaking down the body. You are breaking down a defined structure or area that has been identified as a limitation in order to make the body repair it. You can never just say, "well my hamstrings are tight, so let's get some longer ones to replace mine and then I can touch my toes."

Nope, never gonna happen.

You can never say, "I want to be stronger so I can play professional football," and then head off to the local gym to buy a set of quadricep muscles bigger than yours, put them on and like magic you can run, jump, cut like the best of them.

It takes time, effort, and perseverance, to physically break down your muscles to the point where your body knows that it has to create a rebuilding to make the muscles stronger or more flexible to resist the activity better in the future. We are always trying to make the body more resistance to an activity in the future by exercising. The body wants to be as strong as it needs to be, but no more.

Therefore someone who lacks good core strength and has a hard time controlling their body must do exercises in order to make this area stronger. The entire process however of initiating this strengthening is through a breakdown of the body. This is a hard concept for me to get across at times in the physical therapy clinic.

In order to make the body better we need to break it down.

So therefore we may give an exercise to someone that results in some increased soreness. They may perceive this as a bad thing. After all they are coming in and paying us to take away their pain, not increase it!

Without doing this breakdown process however, we never get the stronger muscle. We would never get the lengthened muscle. The entire premise of physical therapy is breaking down the body for a purpose. It is for this fact that generally most physical therapy diagnoses and problems are worked on for somewhere between 4-8 weeks. That time frame represents the natural physiologic time table that healing is occurring.

It is during this time frame that the rebuild occurs. What you are doing during those weeks however determines what is rebuilt. Your body is going to be what you make it to be. You can let it be the same, or you can create stronger, more capable muscles that now support your joints, and as a result, reduce pain.

The same concept rings true in terms of trying to create range of motion and flexibility within joints and the spaces around the joints. An object at rest stays at rest unless exerted on by an outside force. A tight hamstring will remain a tight hamstring unless acted upon by the person who wants a looser muscle and begins stretching. Seems like a basic concept but it is not usually the first thing you are thinking about when you are in pain.

Most people in pain are acting on the emotions of pain, which generally means they STOP moving!   We get afraid to move. This is why everyone loves the heating pad. It is the comfort food of back pain. There is a positive emotion of "feel good" that comes with the heat and makes them "feel better" emotionally. If the emotion of pain goes down guess what follows? The feeling of physical pain goes down as well. Not unlike overeating on comfort food, the positive emotion effect is only short lived till we are faced with the true problem again. Therefore they may not be able to fully realize the influence the tightness in their body has on their pain.

If you do nothing and allow the pain to dictate what you will do with your body, you will eventually be left with the ability to do less and less. The body will never do more than what you ask it too.

Stretching of the body is a slow process. I had a patient one time equate stretching to cooking barbecue! She said *"So stretching is best done low and slow!"* I said "Yes, you got it!" What she was referring to was making meat very tender (which by the way is muscle) by cooking it at a low temperature over a long period of time. Now back to a real human example: If you take a stretch, and perform it at a low load, over a long duration you will get more stretching of the tissue.

#1 Rule of Stretching: Low load, long duration.

What you bypass by stretching this way is all of the built in internal mechanisms the body has in place for keeping a muscle from stretching too far and tearing. Most people when they stretch, lay back and pull as hard and as far as they can with their leg, arm, whatever. This is absolutely the worst way to stretch. Not only will you activate all the protective mechanisms of the muscle and tendon, you will not get any lengthening as a result.

In the most primitive sense, the body does not know how far you are going to pull the muscle and its only job is top prevent tearing. In a sense it is your body saying it does not trust you to know when to stop stretching! And for the most part, some people can be very thankful this exists. Many patients will say, "Well if I don't feel a good stretch, I don't feel like I'm doing anything." A lot of my time in the clinic is spent educating on the principles of stretching and using them to your advantage.

So we have now talked about how the body is meant to be broken down in order to create a more capable body. This is done through the principles of stretching and strengthening. In the field of physical therapy, there are many other forms of treatment as well and I will touch on them briefly here in the book. This lends a rationale for the basis of the book being a guide for active treatment.

Manual Therapy

I am going to talk about this aspect of physical therapy because it is my specialty, and has the most value when combined with other exercises.

Manual Therapy is the use of what is called mobilization or manipulation of the spine and extremities. It is a "hands on" treatment. I use these treatments everyday, all day. I will have a great deal of people come into my clinic saying "I didn't know you were a chiropractor?" I'm not. I educate them in the utility of manual therapy and talk about the practitioners out there using it. Primarily it comes down to the Doctors of Osteopathic Medicine, Chiropractors, and Physical Therapists.

While each of the practitioners will use manual therapy, only the physical therapist has the true expertise to combine it with exercise for maximal effect. Perhaps this is what makes it so effective in our field. It is the combination manual therapy with exercise that has been shown time and time again to produce the best results.

I will see many patients in my clinic who have been going to the Chiropractor for years, or who have been "cracked" by their D.O. on occasion. I have often thought about "Why are they still having trouble if they have been getting worked on for years?" Maybe it was the wrong techniques, maybe something else.

The overwhelming answer that strikes me is the lack of follow up in the stabilization of joints particularly of the spine following recurrent manipulation. We know based on research studies that the effects of manipulation are good. It can loosen joints, create an improved neurophysiologic flow to the area, decrease muscle spasm, etc. This is why I use these techniques and why other practitioners do them as well. The big issue comes down to the fact that manipulation has only ever been shown to produce *short term* relief and benefit. That means that there was a limit to the effectiveness when only performed in isolation. I can attest to this. In cases where manipulation is the only treatment, it sometimes does not hold up long term. When we correct the joint issues, AND stretch, strengthen, and stabilize the surrounding areas, now we have corrected something for the long haul.

That is what is unique about the physical therapists arsenal. We are the only ones who are going to do this. Some chiropractors will give out exercises, and I have seen physicians give out sheets of things to do, however it does not compare to the depth of the programs we are using in our clinic. I can not speak for all practitioners out there as some are in fact better than others and may be doing things differently, I can only speak to what I have seen clinically.

One thing I should mention very specifically here is that not all Physical Therapists are practicing this way and as a consumer you should seek out someone skilled in the use of these techniques. In my clinic we invest heavily into the training and use of manual hands on skills to use in the treatment of the spine. Some clinicians, from possibly fear or being uncomfortable in treating the spine, may shy away from what we do. This comes back to what I had mentioned earlier in the book where people seem to think of all physical therapy in the commodity realm. It is all the same. Corn is Corn. Oil is Oil.

The people in medicine and chiropractic fields may try to tell you PT is all the same as well. Just not true.

The point is that you can not just go anywhere for physical therapy treatment and expect the same thing. It does not happen. Yes there may be some carryover from certain stretches or strengthening exercises, and that would be great. The problem is that I have seen patients personally who are moving and want to see someone like us where they are moving too and I have to politely say that you are more than likely not going to find it. We are a diamond in the rough.

The best thing to do after reading this book is if you determine the needs of your spine are greater than the stretching routine alone offered in this book, which is sometimes the case, you need to find the best manual therapy practice you can and be evaluated by an expert. If you happen to live in my city or are willing to travel, you are in luck. You can email me at michael.gilbert@gilbertpt.com and we can arrange your visit. Be sure to have your request well written and contact information so we can get in touch with you.

Massage

Massage treatments have been around since the dawn of time. There is evidence dating back to the Greeks, Romans, ancient olympic games, the first physicians and the use of massage for treatment. Many people love the way that a massage feels. There are also many different types of massage. Since I am not a massage therapist, I will not be covering these in full. I bring up the entire idea of massage simply because in the last section of the chapter I was talking about manual therapy. While massage is done manually, I did not include it in the manual therapy section of this book. I did this for the reason that I do not use massage a great deal in my practice.

Some of my colleagues may scoff at the idea that I do not use this and I do not buy into the craniosacral therapies out there, and big myofascial releases that are done. They are in essence forms of soft tissue mobilization with fancy sounding names on top of them. There are a whole host of continuing education seminars out there that will talk about the latest certification practitioners receive to perform the treatment. As it last stands, I have not read many research articles lately that are talking about massage fixing low back pain. I like to keep my practice focused on what is working, and what people need the skill of a therapist for. I am by no means opposed to people going out and getting a massage, it simply is not the best form of treatment for people coming into a physical therapy practice.

For an example, take the person who comes into the clinic with degenerative joints, limited range of motion in the spine, and pain as a result. They describe joints that crack, grind, and "don't sound right" when they are moving. Sound familiar? I find that these are usually the kind of people who do not understand why they have such limitations to begin with. They generally are in mild to moderate pain because the process has come on through wear and tear slowly over the years. They have gradually lost motion over time and therefore never thought of it as a "problem."

These are the type of people who just like to "feel good." They enjoy the aspect of massage because it feels good on their muscles. The biggest problem with this is that degeneration and arthritis are problems with the joints! The joints are what create an effect on the overlying muscles. So a joint that does not move well can cause spasm of the muscle overtop of it. It can create what is also known as a trigger point. A trigger point is a tight ball of contracted muscle that does not easily release and can create pain.

A variety of soft tissue techniques exist to treat these with varying levels of effectiveness. I find that people who work on muscles through the use of massage are often very loud proponents and very defensive about their practices as helpful but not able to back a lot of it with research. That is the problem. We need to know what we are doing is effective. The most effective way to treat joint dysfunctions like arthritis is at the level of the joint. We can not rub out arthritic pain. If we get the joints to move more effectively and therefore put less stress on the muscles, they will automatically stop the spasm and trigger points. Remember these things are reactions to the underlying nervous system as they are stimulated under the surface.

An example I like to give is comparing massaging of muscles for pain control to the flow of water through a hose. Follow me for a minute.

The muscle is the terminal ending point for a nerve that goes from the brain to the muscle. It is also dependent on a bone moving under it. Muscles are present in the body to move and position bones. That is their job. They also act as shock absorbers and joint sensors for position sense. Muscles can have a spasm, become rigid, and have trigger points for a number of reasons, but the main reasons are joints not moving well and over excited nerves. If we rub the muscles or just put some pressure on them on the surface it is no different that having a hose with the water running out the end and you putting your hand on the end to stop the flow of water.

Wouldn't it be a better idea to go back and stop the flow of water at the spigot, which is the source?

I think so.

The minute you take your hand off the end of the hose the water is going to keep flowing. This is the same idea to shut off muscle spasm and trigger points. The underlying joints will continue to stimulate the flow of the spasm to the muscle by sending the signal down through the nerve until the joint has a reason to "shut off."

Why shouldn't we go shut the muscle spasm off at the source? You can not do this by rubbing them. If you massage them, you will temporarily stop the symptoms like putting the hand on the end of the hose, but it will be back. You MUST go back to the joint to shut off the flow.

This is why most people tell me when they got a massage they felt great, but their symptoms came back within a few hours to days. It is because the mode of treatment just does not do what you would like it too. It is passive and involves no movement of your body.

You CAN shut off muscle spasm by working the joints and nerves to produce less muscle tension and spasm. For the person who thinks massage is everything they need for their pain, they need to be reminded that it will never change the underlying structures creating the muscle problems in the first place. You WILL have to at some point address the issue through the joints if you ultimately want to be better.

Massage can be used as an <u>adjunct</u> treatment for the correction of back pain, however should only be used in isolation if the person truly has no internal joint problems and maybe ran too hard in a workout and just needs some lactic acid pushed out of the muscles.

Therapeutic Exercise

This is the bread and butter of the physical therapy approach. This uses the skilled application of various exercises to decrease pain and improve function. There are literally thousands of exercises out there for people to choose from. The trick ends up with choosing the right exercises to go with the right pain and diagnosis.

Getting the *right* exercises is not often achieved with off the shelf type exercise programs with little regard to the mechanics involved. Exercise prescription is also hard to do when given by someone who does not have the necessary pathology knowledge to give the right exercises. What I mean by this is getting some exercises from your trainer, your neighbor, your family, etc. Your family can sometimes be the worst proponent of medical advice out there. Not only are they speaking to you from an emotional standpoint, they may not have very specific knowledge of what they are talking about in the first place and may or may not make you worse off.

I like to talk a great deal in my practice regarding thinking about the "risk" and the "reward" of exercises. In a world where we have so many choices it can be hard to narrow them down. Many people want to do the latest "fad" exercises. They are more exciting to do! I have tons of patients who just get bored with the same old thing. Most people who go to trainers are paying them to come up with these crazy exercise routines that make you feel like "they worked you good!" Is this really good though? Anyone can put someone through an intense workout and make the muscles work hard. Thoughtful application based on the persons orthopedic concerns is totally other subject however.

For example there are many "core exercises" out there. I had a discussion with a patient just the other day about a specific exercise they were doing to strengthen the core. It was a very intense exercise and no doubt worked the core. The problem was they have multilevel degeneration in the spine from the neck down to the lower back. This one exercise alone put a great deal of pressure on the discs of the spine, not to mention irritated the joints and left her in pain for the next two days.

Yes she worked the core.

Yes she could have blown a disc out.

Risk and Reward; was the exercise worth it? I would say not. There would have been countless other ways to work the core that put less pressure on the more important structures of the back. Risk and reward is what we need to be mindful of when coming up with an exercise program.

Exercise is also not JUST about the work of the muscles. You have joints, and capsules, and ligaments, and other structures to be aware of. I think more people would be better served to think orthopedically about exercise than just worrying about taxing the muscles alone. If being treated with physical therapy, you need to make sure your physical therapist is taking an orthopedic approach with you as well.

The next step in exercise selection is about the direction of the movement we choose. We can flex, extend, side bend and rotate our spines. This can be done through a variety of means and can close down joints in one direction, and open them up with the other direction. Knowing what diagnosis is being treated is the first step of choosing the right direction to go. This means we have to do some testing.

An example of this is when someone has a herniated disc, they may benefit primarily from exercise that extends the trunk, while someone with degeneration may benefit mainly from exercises that flex the trunk. It is all about the selection.

So we have now talked about the fact that therapeutic exercise is the cornerstone of physical therapy care. This is what most people associate

PT with. It is also the very thing that may confuse people about doing a physical means of treatment in the first place. Most people can not believe that going to see a PT for their back pain when they can barely move is a wise idea.

How would moving more help, when it already hurts!

Again, it comes down to having a knowledgable practitioner who can "stage" someone for their care. We would not expect someone in acute pain to come in and do jumping jacks. As a matter of fact we expect *no one* to do this. The idea of the PT with the track jump suit training athletes is not what we do. We are skillful at applying techniques to the back and then building it with the correct exercises. This all starts with the exercise selection in the staging process.

I just mentioned the word "staging" of back pain. What is that? Within the scope of exercise selection comes the stage of care someone may be in. Part of our approach to treating back pain is to stage individuals in terms of their pain intensity levels and function. We stage patients one through three when they first arrive for treatment. So if someone comes in for treatment to my practice, they may be in intense pain and not able to move very much. This person would be considered stage one. They are acute, and not going to be a candidate to just jump into exercise. They may need very directed manual therapy techniques in order to decrease their pain, as well as very direct range of motion exercises to help move the spine. Modalities like heat and ice are commonly used in this stage as well, however we will talk about this later in the chapter.

Stage one is also where targeted use of medicine in order to have the person move can be useful. Stage one is the only time I recommend someone use medicine consistently so long as they are using it to help them move! The goal in stage one is to get pain under control and progress the patient to stage two.

Stage two of the treatment phase is also known as the sub-actute phase of treatment. This is the "impairment" stage. Impairments are considered limitations in the body that have adapted over a period of time as a result of pain, life, job, etc. This includes muscle flexibility, muscle strength, endurance and more. Take for example someone that has extreme tightness of the hamstring muscles which are on the back of the thighs. They may have a hard time bending down and reaching for things on the floor. As a result of having this limitation over time, they irritate the back. Thus by stretching and lengthening the muscles that are tight you can reduce the strain on the back and therefore take away pain.

We have people in our practice who are coming directly too us in this stage as well. So the pain is not so severe they can not move, but they are noticing they have day to day trouble with tasks. We are able to do a few more things with this patient compared to someone in stage one because of generally having less pain. In this stage we are commonly strengthening the abdominal muscles of the core as well. We do this in a variety of ways based on the level of fitness of the person in front of us.

People having back pain, who are in stage two, may in fact find the most benefit from this book and the approach presented within. They are generally looking to work the same combination of muscles presented later in the book. By globally loosening the structure they are able to move better and have less pressure on the back. In an enclosed system like the body, having minimal strain is of utmost importance.

Stage Three is the return to work, sport, favorite activity of the person stage of treatment. This is the stage of care where someone is looking to get back to golf, back to work which may require lifting, or work that requires periods of sitting. As a professional treating someone at this point, the focus of care is more situation dependent and giving strategies on how to perform better with the given activity and avoid further injury to the structures of the spine.

I have done a great deal of education in this stage of care regarding the ergonomic set up of one's desk. I have treated a great deal of computer professionals over the years, and each situation has it's own unique challenges. No matter what the challenge however, if a person has trouble with sitting, well then we have to improve the ability to sit! That is a function of flexibility, core strength, posture, and seating surface. If the person is having trouble with lifting boxes and they work for Fed Ex, then we better be working on how to lift the right way and how to prevent further injury.

Stage three encompasses looking at all of these factors, for if we do not treat this way, we are not going to help someone be successful. If I am working with a golfer who has progressed with me through the stages of treatment and has not been back to playing, I have to start doing some golf specific work before putting those demands on the person's body. Golfing can create havoc on the back if not properly trained back into form.

Hopefully what you have taken away from this part of the chapter is that the thought process for selecting exercise tailored to someone's needs is more scientific than what most think. The program I will lay out later in the book takes into account the majority of deficient areas of most person's bodies based on research and clinical practice. We know that the muscle groups mentioned later need to be worked on in the vast majority of cases. It is for that reason the program takes the form it does.

Modalities

What is a Modality? This is a form of passive treatment that is applied to the body in numerous forms and of numerous varieties. Treatments included in this section are items such as heat, ice, electrical stimulation, ultrasound, mechanical traction and iontophoresis. I will cover each of these topics, some more in depth than others. It will not take you long to realize my opinion of these treatments, and where I feel they rank in the spectrum of treatment.

Have you seen a famous professional athlete on TV making a pitch for "Icy Hot?" I have. Visions of Shaquille O' Neil are dancing in my head talking about his back pain and how he could not imagine playing basketball without icy hot. Insert whatever famous athlete you remember and we are in the same place. What the makers of icy hot claim is that the product takes away your pain to help you move again. So how exactly does this work? Does this cream somehow change the mechanical structures of your body? No, it does not. What happens on the surface is the nerve endings that the cream is rubbed over send signals of their own to the brain, therefore disrupting the pain signal being sent at the same time. It is a form of biological scrambling of the signal. This is how a modality works. Since most modalities are passive, they actually do not move any structures (except for traction). The clever people at icy hot however have us convinced we need this cream to push forward. I am guilty, I have used the cream. It was years ago during my football playing days. In a desperate attempt to decrease muscle soreness I remember rubbing it on my body and hoping no one could smell it. If you have ever put it on however, the smell is undeniable. Fact of the matter is that it never took away all the pain, and there is a reason for that. It is not meant to be a cure, just a reliever to help manage. That is the purpose for most modalities, to act as relievers and helpers along the way. We should not think about using modalities in isolation on their own. With all that said, since they are a huge part of our culture and used so widely by everyone, we needed to cover them.

Ice Or Heat?

This is the age old question, and probably the number one question I get from people in pain. If you are reading this book, it is a good bet that at some point in time you have put a hot or cold pack on your back. I have. When you are in pain and no movement is helping and medicine has not made a dent, grab the heating pad and hope for the best, right?

I have been told countless times about someone using a heating pad to fall asleep. This is great except for that some are plugged into the wall! They could be burnt! So we need to be careful. Then there is the moist heat versus the dry heat. There is the ice pack versus the peas in the freezer, versus the ice cup. Many options get debated. Let's talk simply. In the most simple of terms here are the rules for heat and ice:

1. Ice an acute injury, or Ice after activity
2. Heat a chronic Injury, or Heat before activity

The definition of an ***acute injury*** is something that has just happened. This could include a sprained ankle for example. This is the type of injury where you went to lift the box and felt something "wrench" in the back. Sharp, jabbing pain would be the description. This would be the ideal time to put ice on the injury. Inflammation at the area injured can be the reason for the pain. Ice is an ideal way to slow the reaction down.

Heating something that is actively inflamed is going to make the reaction speed up. Think of it like a pot of water. If you want to speed up the water and make it boil and hot, then turn up the heat. If you want to slow the reaction down then you have to cool the water.

The other time you would look to put ice on the injury is after you have gotten done with an activity. Let's say you have been having back pain but you need to help move some boxes. You go and do the activity, experience some pain as a result. This is the time to now lay on some ice.

The definition of a *chronic injury* is something that has been present for a period of time. This includes arthritis, or a nagging back pain that never seems to go away. These types of injuries generally have a good bit of stiffness to go along with them and feel good to heat.

The theory here is that by heating up the tissue we can make it more elastic and therefore make moving easier to do. Now I will say the vast majority of people I treat prefer heat over ice just because it is more comfortable to apply. It also is the most ideal way to prepare the body for movement. Think of a car that is warmed up prior to being driven. The gears move better, the oil lubes the internal parts better and things operate smoother. Same thing in the body. Does externally applied heat do this however to the internal structures? The answer may be different than you think.

Now that we have talked a little about both heat and ice, here is the bottom line. Use whichever feels best if you are not having acute, inflammatory pain. I know I have just presented arguments for both heat and ice. And yes they are both true. But when it comes down to it, both of these treatments for the back are not going to penetrate far enough to influence the discs or nerves. These structures are just too deep and the heat or ice can not get through the barrier of the skin, and muscle tissue to actually bring up the temperature of internal fluid.

Think about it, if heat was able to bring up the internal temperature wouldn't it cause a fever, maybe? I like to give the example of taking a piece of steak, and place a cold pack or hot pack on one side of it. Place your hand on the other side of it. Did your hand get hot or cold? I am not a betting man, but I would have to say no it did not change. Therefore should we expect heat to penetrate in deep and change our backs? Probably not. This is the reason why I say use what feels best if you are not in acute, inflammatory pain. With acute, inflammatory pain always use ice. But if you are in pain and it has been there for a while, use what makes you feel relaxed and better able to move.

The next item to talk about regarding the application of heat or ice is that it is completely passive. Usually you are sitting or lying still with it on. No mechanical movement is happening in the body while it is applied. Sometimes THAT is the reason it makes you feel better, nothing is moving!

We should only ever use these agents to try and promote movement. The main goal of all treatment and full correction is to move. Therefore it is against best practices to advise people to use heat or ice for long term relief of symptoms. More chronic pain has been accomplished by people using these methods of ice or heat to "get by" and never fix the real problems than anything else shy of medicines. Movement is the fix.

In my clinical practice I actually have no hot packs. This may seem tabu for a physical therapy clinic, but I am not in the practice of producing chronic pain. I am utilizing evidence based practice in my clinic for the betterment of the public's health. We know active movement helps people get better faster, and leaves us with less chronic pain.

The last thing I want to promote is putting people in chronic pain. Further, I think in the age of high co-pays and high health insurance premiums it is a travesty to pay someone to put a hot pack on someone. My 5 year old son could do this. A true professional is not needed for this and you should expect more from a treating practitioner.

The take home message here is not that I am against the use of these agents. Ice is *great* for certain injuries. It is usually going to be better for the more superficial (close to the surface) joints. Heat is also good when used correctly. Again, it will be more effective closer to the surface. But use them as a means to help correct the "real" problem by getting active. Do not use them to bandage the problem until the next time, when they may or may not work. Also these things are primarily home remedies, not something someone would need to see a professional about, so expect more from a physical therapist if your pain requires the use of one.

Electrical Stimulation

This form of treatment is also known as TENS (when used for pain control). I speak of this form of electrical stimulation because this is the most popular pain control manner of electric stimulation. Electric stimulation comes in many other varieties as well. It can be for muscle re-education, wound healing, and more.

Electrical stimulation used to be one of the main cornerstones of PT treatment. The process of putting someone on heat and TENS to start treatment or finish treatment with ice and TENS was extremely popular in the field of PT. While this may still exist in some PT circles, we do not do this very often in my clinic. It again comes back to the evidence of what works for the treatment of back pain.

Get people up and moving.

Electrical stimulation gives us an outlet to help someone who may be having a hard time taking medicines due to upset stomach or just not responding to traditional therapies. The electric current is placed on the body via electrodes in a certain manner so as to target an area. There is then a determined amount of electric current that flows through the pads so as to stop a muscle from going into spasm or release a trigger point. It is a direct way to "trick" the brain with a topical form of treatment. There is nothing lasting underneath it. Once the pads come off the reaction will slow and then stop. Again it is a form of treatment that takes our eye off the prize. Our clinical skill is much better served by figuring out the solution to the movement problem than to throw another treatment on that will do nothing more then pacify the symptoms that are being produced. Gotta use it with movement!

Ultrasound

Ultrasound was another cornerstone of treatment and you may have had it if you were in PT years ago. Some people swear by ultrasound.

Others do not think it does anything. Research would side with the group of people who said it did nothing. That is for humans at least. I realize there are a faction of my colleagues out there who will disagree with me on the use of ultrasound. There is a large placebo effect with this treatment. What this means is that in studies where the machine was not even turned on, those people thought they were just as better as the people who actually had the machine on. Yes this has been studied. I mention a lot of times in my seminars I give to the public, that the only studies to have shown benefit for ultrasound were in rat tendons. Since we are humans and not rats, I do not use this treatment, and will not unless some research comes out to show benefit.

Mechanical Traction

Here is the one "modality" treatment that I would recommend for patients. This can be a highly effective form of treatment for herniated discs, lumbar stenosis, disc degeneration, sciatica, etc. Traction is known by a few different names in this day and age. It has been called DTS, decompression, and the more common term for most physical therapy clinics is traction. Chiropractors made popular the DTS and decompression term. This is actually the same treatment as traction. It is also something that is covered by most insurances in the PT world, which is different than the way chiropractors used to advertise for this.

One thing I usually try to educate patients on is that this form of traction that is used today is NOT the same as the traction they may have had in the hospital earlier in life, or that they remembered a family member having earlier in their life. Traction is now done as an outpatient treatment, usually lasting about 15-20 minutes, and is usually always intermittent in nature. Again, it is NOT laying in a hospital bed with weights tied to your body!

The way that the treatment works is a patient can be lying on their back or stomach, and two harnesses are strapped around the patient; one around the chest, and another around the pelvis. The harness is then attached to a computerized head unit, which is then programmed by a physical therapist to apply a traction force to the spine. This is as gentle or as strong as the patient and therapist chooses it to be. The pull is very slow and gradual. It can provide a great way to gap the spaces in the spine to provide space for a nerve to exit the spine with less compression. When a nerve can exit the spine with less compression it means less pain down the legs for a patient.

The treatment of traction can also be used for general loosening of the spine for someone who is dealing with a degenerated disc that simply does not move well. Traction is most beneficial in different positions based on the condition being treated. Disc herniations are different than lumbar stenosis and they respond differently to treatments. You can not treat them the same, and expect good results. Therefore you can not use the traction in quite the same way. This ends up being left to the expertise of the practitioner treating you in terms of how you are placed on the machine, how they set it up, etc.

Something to keep in mind if you are reading this and saying to yourself, "I need traction!" Realize that the main downfall of the treatment is that it is passive. Not unlike the past few modalities we have discussed, we can not solely treat someone with a passive intervention and expect to change the body for the good. We HAVE to use it as a part of a full comprehensive movement program to stretch and strengthen the body. If not used the right way, you may walk away going "this isn't gonna work!"

Like I have mentioned before in the book, buyer beware, you need to realize not all physical therapy is created equal, nor are the people who deliver the care.

CHAPTER 8 KEY POINTS

 Not all physical forms of treatment are the same

 The "side effects" of physical treatment are beneficial to the entire body

 Modalities may offer relief, but not always do what we think they do.

Chapter Nine

What's Your Motivation

I think this is one of ***the most important chapters of the book.*** I say this because until someone has the right "why" to handle and improve their back pain, they will not be successful. I have met many people over the years who during the initial evaluation where I am meeting them for the very first time, the first words out of their mouth are:

" I have been to the surgeon and he says I need surgery to fix my back. I'm not sure how you are going to help me."

"I have tried PT before and I don't think it helped, I'm not sure how you are going to be any different."

"I do not have much hope that there is anything you can do."

Talk about being behind the eight ball right off the bat. There is nothing worse than a pre-conceived notion of something not being effective to ruin your treatment effects. I could put the best treatment plan together ever known to man, but if the person on the other end is convinced it will not work, guess what, it won't.

Psychology of the treatment of back pain is so important that there is what is known as the Fear Avoidance Beliefs Questionnaire used in practice to determine how fearful one is of the back. It can help predict if someone is going to be off work for a period of time and show exactly where their fear about the back lies. Now you may not be sitting there saying you are scared of the back, your feelings may be more skepticism or just lack of faith in the fact that stretching, strengthening, or other treatments conservatively can help you feel better.

No matter what your thoughts are, they ARE going to have an impact in your ability to get better. I have never helped anyone get better who did not believe they could.

The most challenging aspect of practicing in the field of physical therapy is at times walking someone through the mental aspects of having pain. We spend a lot of time and effort to help people learn effective stretching and strengthening in order to change the aspects of their body causing them pain. What is sometimes lost is the mental component. One of the biggest mental components to getting better is doing something long enough to get an effect.

We live in an instant society. You can have anything you want at your finger tips, and at lightning fast speeds these days. Want to watch your favorite show? It's ON DEMAND. We want things NOW. This is no different in the treatment of pain. "My life is busy and I do not have time for this to slow me down." Sound familiar? With all the demands in life, who can take the time to change their body for the long haul to eliminate pain permanently. We opt more often for the quick "fix" to get rid of the pain for now. I have treated patients who have been working on an exercise program for 4-6 weeks and they say, "Well I guess this is not working for me, do I need the MRI or surgery?" I usually follow this by saying, "Hold on, Your pain came from damaging activities over the last 10-20 years and it hasn't reversed in 4-6 weeks?"

Well that can be normal!

People give up fast these days. We are quick to the knife, injection, medicines. What we are slow on is faith of a time tested approach to permanently fix the body.

If you are out there thinking there is no hope, and that nothing can possibly help your back, I challenge you to give the sequence of stretching in this book a try. If you can approach it with an open mind, without pre-conceived ideas, it may lead you to a whole new outlook.

Let's come back to the motivation part of this chapter. This chapter is devoted to the psychology of treating back pain and why it is important to find your own internal "why" for treating your back. Everybody has a different reason they wake up in the morning, go to work, and do whatever it is they like to do. I like to share in the seminars I give that my main motivation at this stage in my life is to be able to keep up with my children and participate in their sports activities and not have pain while doing it! That is why I will continue to do the routine of exercises I came up with 15 years ago for the health of my back today.

Oh, and by the way the routine I came up with is the same routine I am sharing with you in this book! Just in case I forgot to mention that.

Now your motivation may be different than mine. It would be foolish to expect anyone one or two people to share the same specific goal, but in my experience a lot of us want the same things. One of these is to be pain free. For many of my patients they want to keep up with friends and family on trips and not have to be the one slowing everybody down. For others they want to be able to play with their grandchildren without pain. Other people enjoy traveling and need to be able to physically handle hiking, biking, and more.

The common link between all these activities is that they are all examples of "why" someone wants to decrease back pain. A person who can get up in the morning and use the activities as motivation to decrease their back pain will respond much better to treatment than the person who just wishes they had less pain. The person just wishing pain away may have no goal in mind, or they may be too depressed to have their mind focused on what could be possible. So instead of focusing on getting what they want, they simply choose to dwell on the pain and what they can not do.

Ever meet this kind of person. The "Can't Do" person. This is the type of person that no matter what you mention to them, they immediately fire back with a, "Well you can't do that." Or they will put it on themselves, "Well I can't do that because my pain is different than yours." I will also hear things such as, "Well I can't do that because 10 years ago my doctor told me to never let anyone touch my back."

Think about the negative psychological impact that doctor had on that person.

The doctor who gave out that advice was operating on limited knowledge of fields outside of his own and overlooked the benefits of physical therapy. What they effectively did was make that person scared for life to actually do anything physical to help themselves.

The "can't do people" just either *hope* they are eventually going to get better, or there is nothing else out there for them. That type of mentality is a giving up mentality. This book is meant to be the furthest thing from a giving up mentality as you can possibly be.

What I want to spend time on is the "Can Do" attitude and psychology. This is the type of person we all can be if we choose to channel our inner motivation and stay true to it. If you have a big enough <u>why</u>, there is literally nothing out there to stop you from achieving where you want to be.

We are our own self limiting enemies. That little voice inside the subconscious of your mind telling you that you can not get there. That whatever treatment you are doing wont work. *You can sabotage your own results!* This type of thinking may ring true more for someone who is dealing with or has dealt with chronic pain in the past or present time. If you constantly convince your mind that something will not work, then guess what, there is a good chance it will not work. If you consistently train yourself to be positive and focused on the building and continual effort to get better and the "why" you want to get better, I will undoubtedly say you will reach your goal of getting better.

Let's explore this one step further. I have been on the receiving end many times of a person who I have just started to treat, or who I have seen for a few visits. Then, all of a sudden they just decide they have not seen the results they are looking for and they decide to stop coming in for treatment. They essentially give up just after starting!

Sometimes what forces them to stop is the initial discomfort, which they are fearful of, from starting to stretch muscles that have not been used in a while. They just can't see how moving more is going to help decrease their pain. They begin to rationalize their pain as something they just have to accept and live with because they tried to help it and things only got worse. Ever hear the " Well if I just don't go up stairs I'm fine with everything else." That is rationalizing pain at its finest.

The worst thing in the world for folks who are fearful of pain is anything reminiscent of pain coming back. They may have had a bad previous experience with trying to get moving. Many people have already spent time in the past trying to get their pain down to the point "they could live with. " It is a huge red flag for them if your initial program of movement makes them worse. Their motivation gets ruined at the start.

The whole notion of just getting to where you "could live with the symptoms" to me is a cop out from where you truly can get to and deserve to be. Most of the people in this situation HAVE tried dealing with back pain in the past and have been treated with physical therapy before as well. These are people who are not averse to trying stretching. They simply have mentally convinced themselves they can not get better.

On the surface, they tell you they WANT to get better, but then their actions prove different. If there is one truth I can tell you, it is that you CAN NOT take away years of degeneration in 20 days. You can not do it in 40 days. You can make strides along the way, but it is impossible to have true change in the body faster. The body repairs and builds itself through a process of breakdown. ***Without going through the breakdown first, you can never get the body to start the buildup process.*** It is the lack of someone wanting to <u>feel</u> some of the breakdown that ultimately never allows them to reach the build up process.

Now I am not trying to pick on this, but I will tell you it is the one biggest mental and physical hurdle I see people have to get by when they have dealt with pain in the past. If you think surgery is the only way, and you are afraid to let go and have faith in the conservative healing process, then you have a big barrier in front of you. This is the person who would rather rely on shots for the back because it gives them more time to keep doing what they want to do without truly addressing the problems in the back. To the person who is using the shots as a spring board to take care of the mechanical problems, congrats to you, you are the exception to the rule.

I will liken decreasing pain to weight loss, which is something most of us in our lives have tried to do. In our country we have a tremendous amount of diets, diet centers, and plans for people to follow, yet we are also becoming more obese at a faster rate than ever.

If all the diets worked, and everyone followed them we would be in a better place, right? Well it is the brain that needs convincing. Motivation to stay the course is vital.

Diets and exercise are easy. It is convincing yourself to do it that is hard. We like things instantly. If we do not see the pounds coming off after 14 days of eating lettuce, I do not know too many people who will just keep eating lettuce. They fall off the wagon, go back to what they always have done, and hope something else pops up along the way. What happens? No weight loss, that is for sure. The same thing goes for pain and using a physical means to treat it. If the back hurts, and someone does a stretching program and feels no better, then they are not likely to do it in the future. If the positive feedback does not happen fast, what is the motivation to continue?

Just because a stretch doesn't work instantly, does not mean you throw it away yet. Is that an extremely tight area of your body? Have you neglected that area for months or years? Could it be **THE** limiting factor in you crossing the abyss to finally resolve your pain?

Giving up on physical treatment at that moment can be the difference between continuing the life long struggle of up and down pain symptoms, or full long term back pain resolution. Some of this comes down to motivation and trust. If you do not have full faith that you can get there, or in the person instructing you, it can be a huge barrier ultimately in whether or not you are going to get better.

I am a huge believer in the fact that whatever you think you can achieve, you can. An author named Napoleon Hill has echoed this statement in many success oriented books. The inverse of this is true as well. If you do not think you can get there by doing exercise, then I bet you won't. You have to make the decision for yourself.

I have seen people who I would have never thought they could get better, achieve outstanding results. I have seen someone after back surgery and multiple fusions of the spine ski again for the first time in 20 years.

That person not only felt that the exercise program could work, they are now addicted to the exercises rather than the pain pills! Awesome side effects of exercise!

Did this person get there in 20 days...NO. Does everyone want that result in 20 days, YES. If you truly want to get better, get your mind right and then start executing the little things. The results over time are tremendous. Following the stretching program outlined in this book is a great tool. It could be just the beginning for you however. If you can control back pain, then it serves as a spring board to more activity.

I have spent a great deal of attention here on how internal motivations personally help control back pain, however back pain is also a larger issue than just one person. We can talk about creating motivation to improve health within companies and improve work related tasks. Employee motivation to keep working through back pain is very important to employers out there. What if your livelihood was at stake because of your back pain? What if you lost your business because of back pain?

The person or company employing other people has a great deal of motivation to have their employees healthy and free of back pain. Back pain is one of the leading causes of loss of work and costs the labor industry. The Institute of Medicine has estimated that the annual value of lost productivity due to pain in 2010 dollars ranged between $297 billion and $335 billion. Yes that was Billion, with a B. If you are a business owner, I think those figures are reason enough to get all of your employees doing this grouping of exercises recommended in this book.

You can compute your own lost earnings as a company due to the effects of back pain. The nursing and trucking industries are two of the largest occupation groups for back pain. My clinic is located near a US Navy base. These folks are encouraged to exercise at work and even have some time built in to exercise. That is great! This book could give further guidance on how to use that time more efficiently in order to get a definite return on the time they are investing.

The motivation for someone who is out of work with back pain is a delicate one. On one end you can have people who try to use the back as an excuse to remain out of work, and on the other hand you can have someone who is genuinely not able to do the work they need to do, or love to do in order to make a living. How do you know what is the motivation for one?

Since work for most people is a Monday - Friday proposition, the "why" factor can be quite a big reason for getting better (or not getting better!). If they do not like working, there is not much "why" to get better. There is a term out there called a malingerer. This is a person who purposefully "milks" a condition for all they are worth in the avoidance of going back to work. This can be extremely frustrating from the employer end due to the fact that they in most cases NEED someone on the job that person was hired to do.

Now the effectiveness of this book on people who genuinely have no interest in getting better is going to be minimal. Someone has to have some starting motivation to get better in order to get results from this book. Luckily, people really do not like to be in pain. Furthermore most people are not acting like they are in pain for attention. Yes there are a few. For the most part however, I believe the majority of people are truly interested in getting better.

Now that we have discussed the different motivating factors that are involved in getting better it is time for you to write down your motivating factors.

What is it that makes YOU want to get better?

Get out your pen or pencil and write down your top 5. This does not have to be an exercise that takes you more than 5 minutes. Do not overthink the reasons. They should be very everyday and obvious to you. Write down below the 5 reasons you want to improve the health of your back:

....

....

....

....

....

Now take these reasons that you have written above and do something within the next 24 hours to influence them for the positive. That could mean flipping to the next chapter and diving into the exercises to help the health of your back.

It could mean more than just exercise for the back. It could mean taking a look at your time management so that you can fit the program into your daily routine. It could mean taking a look at your diet and more.

The point is the quicker you take action on what you just wrote down the more likely you are to follow through on it. Do not just read the book to this point and not do anything further. Do not keep wasting time if you are having pain. Get rid of it. Start the process now and stick with it. Prove to yourself that you can follow through on a series of stretches. It is not that hard, you just have to "do it" as Nike says.

CHAPTER 9 KEY POINTS

 You need to find your own motivation

 The "Why" you are doing the exercises are just as important as the exercise itself

 Start within the next 24 hours to take action

Chapter Ten

The Formula:
The Gilbert Sequence

So up to this point in time we have talked about a lot of components that come into play for the successful treatment of back pain. I have told you about the fears and worries associated with back pain, the way my profession of physical therapy helps back pain, the anatomy of the spine, and how motivation is a huge factor in whether or not someone gets better.

It is now time to get into the meat and potatoes of the book, and that is the actual sequence of stretches that can ultimately shape your back for the future. This sequence of exercises is not rocket science. It CAN however, provide quite dramatic effects on the back. This is a series of exercises that has been done, tested, and proven time and time again to work. How can I make such a claim? Well, I lived it. It is also what I use to help thousands of people with back pain over the past 10 years. This is the exact routine I used to beat 3 herniated discs in the low back, constant sciatica, and little to no participation in life. Here are the list of things I have done SINCE herniating 3 discs in the lower back 15 years ago.

1. Dead lifted 450 pounds
2. Squatted 400 pounds (with a straight bar on the back)
3. Ran 2 Half Marathons
4. Participated in Olympic Weightlifting
   1. Clean and Jerk 250 pounds
   2. Snatch 185 pounds. (these are not earth shattering weights for people who REALLY do this, but for a guy with a bad back, not too shabby!)
5. Ran Multiple 5K and 10K events
6. Many Rounds of Golf
7. Became a jungle gym for my kids to play on!
8. Too many others to keep going!

The point here I am trying to make is that life after a back problem, can keep going. It is all in how you lay the foundation for the back that will influence what it will become. We all want the back that just gets up in the morning and works. The fact of the matter however is that in order to achieve this, you have to do the work first. This is a plant the seed and then reap the harvest type of thing. You can never harvest the seed you have not planted.

The next point I would like to make as we begin this chapter is that the sequence matters! Yes, the muscles will loosen systematically through this approach. It is therefore my recommendation that you do the exercises in order. That means do them the same way every time. Do not try to get fancy, do not try to make them more than they are. If you can not feel the stretch in the way you think you should, you very well may have perfectly fine flexibility in that muscle group. Do not overly loosen this area. The body is meant to work in certain length - tension relationships. It is the goldilocks phenomenon. The porridge being not to hot, not too cold, just right. Well in the body, muscles work best when not too tight, not to long.

More often than not, we look at the dancer or gymnast with great flexibility and think to ourselves, "Boy I wish I could do that." "They must have no pain at all." Wrong. I will typically see these people after they are done competing usually for pain related to hypermobility, or better known as <u>too much</u> movement. The reason they develop pain is because when they were competing they were very strong through a large range of motion. The body was constantly being worked. Now enter the REAL world of sitting at a desk or in a car and they no longer are working their bodies quite as hard. The range that they used to have in their muscles typically remains, but the strength to control the range goes way down. This is the opposite problem of someone having too little movement. For this type of person they may need something other than a stretching routine to get well, they may need a stability program. I am not saying this approach will not work for you if you are an overly flexible person, but realize if too much movement is your problem, you can not only do stretches to get better, you must strengthen as well. If you are generally tight muscle wise, than this sequence is right up your alley.

Now, I do not expect you to have tightness in *ALL* the muscle groups this sequence of stretching goes through. You should not expect this either. Most people's bodies are not train-wrecks of tightness, but have key areas of tightness that over time wear down a very specific area and therefore create pain around the structures effected. I want you to make sure that you take advantage of your natural strengths, and bring the weaknesses up to speed.

I mentioned just a moment ago that it is usually the surrounding structures of a tight area creating the pain in the body. I say this because when is the last time you felt your disc? I hate to say it, but I am all but going to guarantee you have no idea what it is like to feel your disc. When is the last time you felt muscle pain? Joint Pain? Now were talking. Most of you know what these areas feel like. These are the structures we are after. They are the ones that when influenced, take the pressure off of disc and nerves. Influencing these structures is how you take away sciatica, back pain, and how you get back on the path of activity.

The Sequence

This is the exact method I used for the successful resolution of pain coming from herniated discs in my OWN lower back. I have used these same exercises for the successful relief of numerous diagnosis in my clinic. If you suffer from any of the following, this routine is for you:

1. Herniated Discs
2. Arthritis
3. Stenosis
4. Degenerative Disc Disease

5. Sacroiliac Dysfunction
6. Piriformis Syndrome
7. Sciatica
8. Scoliosis
9. And More....

The previous diagnosis list is to be used as a guide and is not all inclusive. Will there be certain limitations and restrictions within each of these diagnoses? Yes, there will be, no two things are quite the same. No two people are the same either, and what works for Joe down the street may not work the same for you. Here is my disclaimer that while the vast majority of people are going to have success with this program, do not despair if it does not work for you. A few things to consider. One, you must see the process through (see the challenge chapter in this book!). Two, you can not expect instant results. Remember that the instant fix is not real. I have full faith that if you commit to the basics of this approach, it will help your back. Now let's dive in.

Exercise #1

Single Knee to Chest

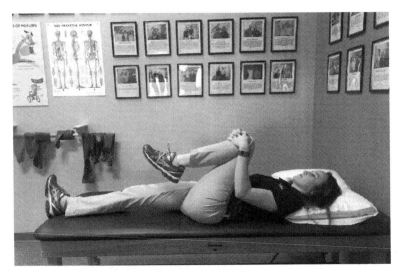

Figure: Single Knee to Chest (SKTC)

This exercise in the first step in the sequence. It is designed to be completed laying flat on your back. It can be done on the floor, on the bed, on a yoga mat, etc. Just complete the exercise somewhere that is comfortable for you to lay on your back. During this exercise you will be pulling one of the knees up toward the chest while the opposite leg remains flat. This will stretch the glute muscle and the upper hamstrings on the side of the leg that is being pulled toward the chest.

This stretch will also be "opening" the spacing of the lower back on the side of the pulling. It is for this reason it is a good stretch for opening the space known as the foramina. This then allows the nerves more room to exit the spinal canal and travel down the legs. When this space is open, there is less pressure on the nerve and therefore less pain as a result of the nerve being compressed.

The stretch is held for a period of 30 seconds, and repeated 3 times in a row on one side before switching to the other side. The reason for completing all stretching on one side before going to the next is to maximize the amount of elongation of the muscle and joint. When you compound the stretching in this manner, the stretch is allowed to build as you go rather than constantly switching back and forth which allows the tissues on one side of the body to rebound back while you stretch the other side.

An alternative to this stretch for someone who has pain with keeping the opposite leg laying flat is simply to bend the knee that is not being pulled back. This will help to take some pressure off of the lower back.

Exercise #2

Piriformis Stretch with a Push

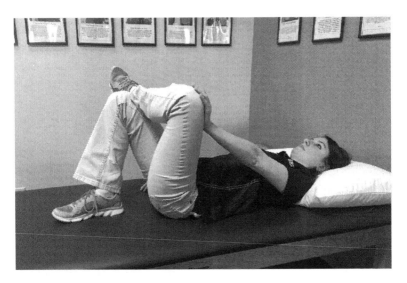

Figure: Piriformis with a Push

The next exercise in the sequence is known as the piriformis with a push. I chose to do this exercise next in the sequence because of the flow from the single knee to chest into this one. This exercise is started in the same position as the single knee to chest. You will start with both legs in the bent position. You will be laying flat on the back. Next, cross one leg over the other without trying to bring the stationary (noncrossed leg) closer across the midline. This essentially will look like you are putting the ankle on the opposite knee.

Once the leg is crossed you will feel a pulling/ twisting of the hip joint and buttock of the leg being turned. Take the hand on the side of the knee and give a slight push forward on the knee. You will feel a greater intensity of the stretch, but at the same token, you are not trying to stretch too far. Listen to you body, for it will let you know when the intensity of the stretch is too much. If you push too hard, you will also be engaging the internal mechanisms of the body to actually fight the stretch and prevent the stretch from being effective. This is a great stretch that will work the pirifomis muscle which has a direct ability to compress the sciatic nerve or limited the motion of the hip therefore effecting the mechanics of the pelvis. The stretch also works on loosening the joint capsule of the hip.

The stretch is held for a period of 30 seconds, and repeated 3 times in a row on both sides. Again, this is a stretch where you want to complete all the stretches on one side before moving to the other side.

The piriformis muscle can be stretched in other ways as well. It is not my intent to actually teach you all the different ways to stretch this muscle in this section of the book but to just make you aware there are more varieties than the one I am presenting to you. This manner in which I am instructing in the book is designed to work both the muscle as well as the joints in the surrounding areas. That is the reason I have choose this one. Others practitioners may like to do the other variety and that is their choice.

Exercise #3

Prone on Elbows

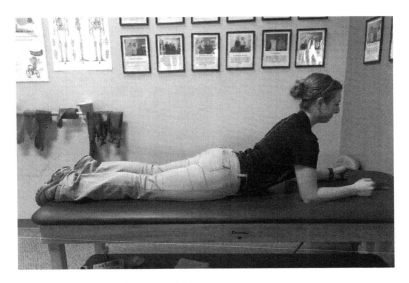

Figure: Prone on Elbows Position

Continuing on in the sequence is the exercise of prone on elbows. This one is actually counterintuitive mainly because it is really no exercise at all. It is a positional hold where you will roll to your stomach after completing the piriformis with a push. So there is no net movement with this exercise.

The main purpose of this exercise is to restore some of the lordosis to the lumbar spine. The term lordosis is the name given to the curvature of the spine in this region. For a good number of people who are suffering from degeneration, loss of lordosis can create a flattening of the spine and make it hard to stand upright. Also people who constantly sit at a desk are going to have adaptive shortening of the muscles on the front of the trunk and a molding of the spine into a flexed position over time. Getting the spine in the opposite position is needed to remold the spine for proper weight bearing.

During this prone on elbows exercise pictured you want to roll to the stomach and prop up onto your elbows just as if you were going to be watching TV in front of you. You will maintain this position for about one minute. You are *not* going to repeatedly extend up, just maintain the position. That's it! Easy exercise.

This exercise is not to be confused with a McKenzie exercise. While these exercises can be effective for some, there is a grouping of patients who should not be using McKenzie based exercises which are nothing more than repeated extension exercises. Before the McKenzie people ridicule that statement, we should all realize that most people in the public associate Mckenzie with repeated extension of the spine.

The main issue with these exercises is that they will close down the facet joints on the back of the spine and pinch down on nerves in a spine which is degenerated or has stenosis. The approach works well for herniated discs, but you really need a evaluation by a physical therapist to determine if the exercises are a good fit. In a classification system of treatment for the lower back, extension based exercises only make up 25% of the grouping. Some people are going to be home runs, others will have a disastrous experience. Do not just blindly follow McKenzie exercises because your neighbor did well with them or because you had a "McKenzie trained therapists" prescribe them. The McKenzie therapists pay good money for a certification that pigeon holes the thought process more than helps in my opinion. My McKenzie trained colleagues who took the time to learn it will not like those words. I took the courses as well. Decided not to be certified. Realize all PT's are trained in McKenzie principles, some parts of the country are just more enthralled with it than others. I happen to practice in a part of the country/my home state that thinks it is the "be all end all" of back pain treatment. I politely disagree with that notion.

Exercise #4

Hip Flexor Stretch

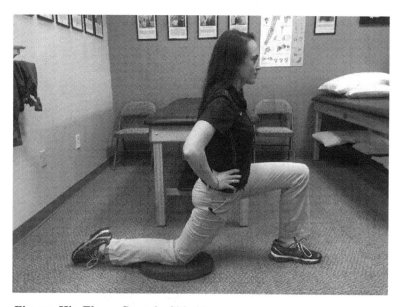

Figure: Hip Flexor Stretch: Side View

The next stretch in the sequence is to stretch a muscle known as the hip flexor or "groin". This is a group of muscles comprised of the psoas and the iliopsoas muscles. The big reason to stretch these muscles is because of the direct connection they have to the spine and the lower extremity.

For a lot of people these days, jobs can be very sedentary in nature an lead to long periods of time sitting in front of a computer. Think about all of the cumulative build of time spent in the seated position over the course of life for someone working at a desk 8 hours a day, 5 days a week and for 30 years! That is a lot of time spent in one position over the years and this results in adaptation of the muscle over time into a shortened length. This would cause trouble with standing fully upright when getting out of a chair, or problems with having a full and normal stride length during walking.

It is for the above stated reasons that this exercise is the next most important in the sequence of exercises. When being done, the stretch is best completed down on a knee with the other foot out in front. In this "split stance" the body will be translated forward, but not so far that the front knee would go over the toes.

The stretch should be felt on the front of the hip and thigh of the **back** leg which will be down on a pillow or cushion. It is possible to feel it in other places, however you want to focus on feeling a pulling sensation on the front of the thigh. The stretch should be held for 30 seconds and repeated 3 times in a row all on one side first, and then it can be switched to the opposite side.

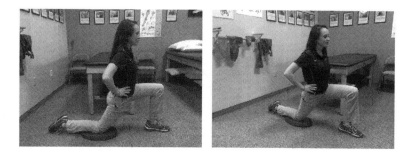

Figure: These show the correct way to perform the hip flexor stretch. Note the back is not arched or flexed forward, and knee does not go over the toes.

The caution with this exercise is for people who have problems with the knee. If you have a knee problem or replaced knee which makes it hard to kneel down there are alternatives. You can perform a similar exercise by laying on the back at the side of a bed. One knee is pulled up to the chest and the other leg is allowed to hang over the side of the bed. Just make sure you do not fall off!

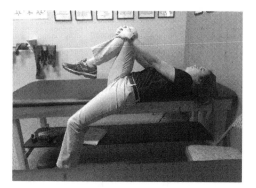

Figure: Alternate Hip Flexor Stretch if you have problems on your knee. Make sure the surface you are on is stable.

Exercise #5

Hamstring Stretch

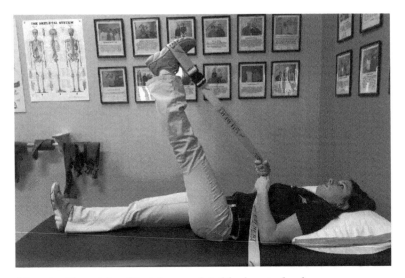

***Figure: Hamstring Stretch completed laying on back
with a stretching strap***

The hamstring stretch in my opinion is one of the most important
stretches for the lower back. Not only is it tight for most people, it is
one of the most pain generating areas of the body when someone lacks
flexibility there. When someone has sciatica, this is the muscle that
most people are going to feel the effects in. The sciatic nerve runs

right down along the hamstring muscle. When you bend down to pick something up, you are stretching the hamstrings. When you bend down to put socks and shoes on, you are stretching the hamstring muscles. So these muscles have to perform well or they can pull on the back in a painful manner at all points in the day, all day long.

Can you touch your toes? No prize for this by the way, but if you can not touch your toes you may have tight hamstrings! Now let me be very clear, the ability to touch your toes has no bearing on whether or not your back can get better. In fact, in my opinion one of the worst ways in the world to stretch the hamstrings is to just bend over. Yes you will stretch them, and yes you will feel a pull in the back of the thighs, but you will also be sending the pressure of the discs in the spine through the roof and you are liable to blow a disc out!

The hamstring stretch is performed with the same count as the previous stretches. You would pull the leg up being stretched while keeping the other flat. If you have to, you can bend the leg that is flat on the table for comfort. Ideal position is flat however. The stretch leg should be held 30 seconds and then repeated 3 times in a row on the same leg before going to the next leg. You only have to break for a few seconds between the sets, just enough to give your hands a break.

I know I have mentioned it before, but the following advice warrants repeating. There is risk and reward with all exercises. Our job is to place someone at the least amount of risk for the most amount of reward with a given exercise/ stretch. The rewards of doing a stretch correctly can virtually ensure that you are on the way to having a successful outcome in treating your back pain.

So there you have it. I have presented to you the 5 exercises that will take you about 20 minutes to complete. You should actually be able to finish in even less time than that. In total there is 780 seconds of stretching. To give you an idea, there are 1,200 seconds in 20 minutes. If we do quick math (20 min = 1200 seconds - 780 seconds of stretching = 420 seconds left over). The 420 seconds gives you plenty of time for breaks between sets, 7 minutes to be exact. So get going and you will be done in no time.

To end this chapter I would like to reinforce on a topic I can not **over**emphasize enough. In order to truly benefit and have improvement with this routine you have to have the right mindset and expectations. There will be some of you who do this routine and hit a home run and have less pain almost instantly. Great! For the rest of you it will be about putting one foot in front of the other and slowly chipping away at your pain. This can be for a number of reasons, some of which has entirely to do with where your current level of fitness is and how far up the mountain you have to climb. The other reason is simply that most good things in life take time to build and your body is no different. You get out what you put in.

Do this routine daily and the compound effect over time will begin to change your body and as a result your pain. If you chose to start the process and give up or get distracted along the way you can always get back on track with the philosophy that tomorrow is a new day and the start of the rest of your life. You get to chose how each day is going to start and how you handle the adversities that come with each one.

So if you miss a day, who cares! Don't beat yourself up.

Get back in the saddle tomorrow and get it done. If you follow through, you will be successful. Small gains over time are laying the foundation for a life of being able to use and abuse the back without the fear of it crumbling. You only get one back (no replacements here folks), treat it well.

At the end of this chapter you will find a "daily progress report" you can use to track your progress with the stretching routine. In the clinic we record exercises for a purpose; that purpose is so we know they are done! The daily progress note will let you keep track of the stretching you did, or make notes as to why you did not do them that day. Write down in the notes section what stretches you struggled with on a given day. Write down the day you noticed a stretch getting easier. Write down how your back felt that day so you can compare along the way (this will help with the challenge coming up!). Nice part is by the time you are done with this program you more than likely will need no reference of the progress reports because everything will be committed to memory.

If you have trouble with any of the exercises, check out our demonstration videos at our you tube channel for Gilbert Physical Therapy. There is a link to the channel on our website **www.gilbertpt.com**.

CHAPTER 10 KEY POINTS

🔑 Do you understand the sequence of exercises?

🔑 Realize that true change takes time and effort.

🔑 Remember the Compound Effect

🔑 When will you start....How about now!

20 Min Back Pain Solution
Daily Progress Report

Date: ....

Start Time: .... Finish Time: ....

Day .... of 90

Exercise	Time and Repitions	
	Right	Left
Single Knee to Chest		
Piriformis with a Push		
Prone on Elbows		
Hip Flexor Strech		
Hamstring Strech		

Notes for the Day: ....

....

....

....

....

Chapter Eleven
Conclusion

As I write the conclusion to this book, I am grateful for having the experiences in life I have had. At the moment that I was dealing with back pain I would not have said the same things! But from that experience, I developed the desire to help others. I am grateful for the ability to pass along this information to you.

I take great pride in the fact that you have read this far and hope that you found the book entertaining, informative, and walk away with some kind of energy and enthusiasm for making your back better. I know that after reading this book you will have a renewed spirit in the sense that back pain does not have to ruin and take away your quality of life. Whether you are pursuing an athletic endeavor, or just want to walk around the block and play with your kids or grandkids you can benefit from this book.

It does not matter if you are 30 years old or 80 years old. This book is your guide and can help you.

The other final thought I want to leave you with is that this book is also just the beginning. If you are truly into fitness or have a desire to perform at a higher level, this book would literally just break the ice.

The world of strengthening, especially for the back is so diverse and broad that we would need an entirely new book to cover the scope. There are so many opinions out there.

For the folks out there reading this who are interested in treatment on another level, see my offer at the beginning of this book. I am available for individual appointment via emailing **michael.gilbert@gilbertpt.com.** I chose email even though the amount of junk and spam email I already receive is already over the top. At last check I currently have over 14,000 unread junk emails. None the less email is extremely easy and accessible to everyone. I am willing to work with you whether you are an elite athlete, corporate executive, or retired grandma down the street. The beauty of this approach is that everyone can benefit from a physical means of treatment.

Chapter Twelve
The Challenge

In the preface to this book I mentioned that I started writing this book as just an information based book with the goal of hoping to transform the lives of people with back pain. I was hoping my message would inspire people to improve the health of their bodies and decrease their pain! During the process however I could not help but continue to think about ways I could make people actually go from just reading this information and hearing about my story to really fully embracing the information and doing something about it. Then it hit me.

Shortly after I went through my own back pain and came through the other side I wanted to push further. I had completed this sequence of exercises and improved the health of my back to become more mobile and strong, so I decided to take a challenge on myself.

The name of the challenge was called Body For Life. As an avid lifter I was intrigued by the transformation challenge as it was halfway between bodybuilding and more of a realistic "everyday joe" chance for competing and getting in better shape. I had friends through college who were extremely athletic and into body building and had arguably a much better ability to do the "real" bodybuilding, so this route appealed more to me. At this point in life I wanted to recoup the strength and fitness I lost through inactivity following back problems. For those of you out there who have never heard of Bill Phillips or read the book Body For Life, I highly recommend it. Bill Phillips created the challenge for these ordinary people to become extraordinary. I do not know Bill personally, but still feel respect for him for the challenge he introduced. The results were fabulous and many people had positive changes in their lives because of that challenge.

Following my back problem I was left with some unwanted weight I felt the need to lose that accumulated over the months of being inactive and unable to move. I completed my challenge in the following 12 weeks after my back injury. I finished lean, in great shape, and felt on top of the world. I did not win the competition. But I got every bit out of the competition as I thought I would have. My back was not hurting, I was strong and could do more athletically than I ever have.

The other nice part about the challenge was that it was not just about how you looked. It was also about the mental changes and challenges you overcame. That was half the judging. There were great prizes given away. Even though I walked home with no prize, I actually felt fine with that for the way my body felt was the prize. So as I wrote this book, I kept having flashbacks to the challenge *mentality* and the way I felt energized to compete and follow through on my commitment. I could not help but feel that would be a great way to get people involved in their "want" to get rid of their back pain. So much of back pain is mental as well as physical.

With all that you have learned in this book (the right motivation and a sequence of exercises at your disposal proven to work) I would like to issue **YOU** a challenge.

Now yes, this will be different from a "true fitness" challenge. This is not a weight loss challenge or strength gain challenge. *This is a back pain elimination challenge.* This is a life changing, reclaiming challenge.

I believe you can have a pain free back and full life. For the next 90 days, which is roughly 3 months I challenge you to perform the above sequence of exercises for no more than 20 minutes per day. If you are willing to take the time to do this, I believe you can have the pain free back you hope for and desire. More people are out there dealing with back pain than you think. Back pain is extremely limiting to daily life. It cost companies hundreds of thousands, if not millions of dollars annually in sick time and workers compensation.

If you are a CEO, company president, business owner, whoever you are, challenge your employees. Have them read this book as required reading. Give them a discount on health insurance if they do. If they perform the challenge I will bet you will have less sick time and workers compensation claims to deal with. A healthy back is an asset rather than a liability.

Who else can you think of who should take this challenge?

Maybe a loved one, a friend, colleague, neighbor? If you are going to embark on improving your own back, nothing makes more sense than having someone else do it with you!

The diet industry has done this forever. So no different here. Have them read the book as well. Let them be convinced to start doing this stretching routine with you. The only thing they have to lose is less pain! If you are going to lose all of your pain, make them lose theirs as well so they can keep up with you!

Write down the people in your life who need this help here:

....

....

....

....

....

Give them a copy of the book. Take them on the journey. I am excited for you to start. Do not be discouraged if you do not feel all your pain go away right away. This is the exception to the rule. To have true pain elimination you have to change from the inside out and this takes small steps over time. Doing the routine over the next 90 days is what will enable you to make this change happen. Your body will have the time to adapt. Focus on the week to week and month to month changes, not the day to day. We all want instant gratification. If you do, this approach is not for you and more than likely you will never get to where you truly want to be. You must have a strong enough "why" to do this and stay focused on it. If you do, you can kiss your back pain goodbye.

Good luck!

Make sure to share your success story with us at **www.gilbertpt.com**. Fill out the "contact us" form and let us know about your success. Don't forget to follow us on Facebook as well.

Like us at **www.facebook.com/GilbertPT.**

Biography

Michael M. Gilbert, DPT

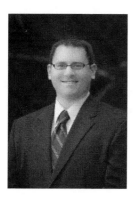

Dr. Michael M. Gilbert, DPT (Doctor of Physical Therapy) was born and raised in Harrisburg, PA. Upon graduating high school Dr. Gilbert earned a bachelors degree in Kinesiology with a medical emphasis from The Pennsylvania State University.

Dr. Gilbert earned his Doctor of Physical Therapy degree from the University of Pittsburgh. During training Dr. Gilbert completed multiple internships specializing in treatment of the spine along with a host of other orthopedic conditions.

Dr. Gilbert has worked in many settings over the past 10 years with outpatient orthopedics being his preferred area of expertise. He has worked during training in the UPMC center for sports medicine alongside the Pittsburgh Steelers and Pirates facilities. Beyond that Dr. Gilbert has attended many continuing education classes on the spine with a primary focus on the manual hands on treatment of the spine. He is a member of the American Physical Therapy Association, The Orthopedic Physical Therapy Association, and a Member of the Private Practice Section.

Dr. Gilbert established Gilbert Physical Therapy in 2012 with his business partner Chad Madden. Since then, Gilbert PT has been able to enhance the lives of many people who have struggled with back pain and other conditions. We have quickly become the leader in central PA for the treatment of back pain.

Dr. Gilbert hosts monthly back pain seminars/workshops for the public and speaks extensively around the area on back pain. He has been featured on local TV educating the public on various topics in physical therapy. Dr. Gilbert is always open to new speaking opportunities and can be reached at **michael.gilbert@gilbertpt.com.** Please send an email request if you would like to have Dr. Gilbert speak to your group or facility.